UNIVERSITY OF
WOLVERHAMPTON

The —

The Contact Lens Manual
A practical fitting guide

Andrew Gasson FBCO, DCLP, FAAO
Contact Lens Practitioner, London, UK
and

Judith Morris MSc, FBCO, FAAO
Director, Institute of Optometry, London, UK

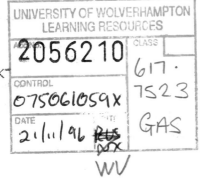
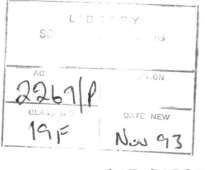
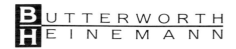

BUTTERWORTH
HEINEMANN

Butterworth-Heinemann Ltd
Linacre House, Jordan Hill, Oxford OX2 8DP

PART OF REED INTERNATIONAL BOOKS

OXFORD LONDON BOSTON MUNICH
NEW DELHI SINGAPORE SYDNEY
TOKYO TORONTO WELLINGTON

First published 1992
Reprinted 1992

British Library Cataloguing in Publication Data
Gasson, Andrew
  The contact lens manual: A practical fitting guide.
  I. Title   II. Morris, Judith
  617.7

ISBN 0 7506 1059 X

Library of Congress Cataloguing in Publication Data
Gasson, Andrew.
  The contact lens manual : a practical fitting guide / Andrew
  Gasson and Judith Morris.
  p.   cm.
  Includes bibliographical references and index.
  ISBN 0 7506 1059 X
  1. Contact lenses.   I. Morris, Judith.   II. Title.
  [DNLM: 1. Contact Lenses.   WW 355 G254c]
  RE977.C6G38 1991
  617.7′523–dc20
  DNLM/DLC   91–13545
  for Library of Congress   CIP

Composition by Scribe Design, Gillingham, Kent
Printed and bound in Great Britain by Redwood Press Ltd, Melksham, Wilts

Contents

Foreword

There are probably around thirty contact lens textbooks currently available in the English-speaking world. These books are generally biased towards the particular interests of the author, which may be, for example, medical, technological or pathophysiological. In addition, some textbooks concentrate on specific topics such as rigid or soft lens fitting. So why another contact lens textbook?

The authors of this book, Andrew Gasson and Judith Morris, are clinicians who have achieved eminence in this field via lecturing and writing on the real practicalities of contact lens fitting. They have pooled their ideas and experiences into this textbook which will stand alone amongst the others – for this book is about practical, clinical, hands-on contact lens fitting.

For detailed physiological discourses on the ocular response to lens wear, or physico-chemical analyses of contact lens materials, the reader will need to go elsewhere. For a thorough, direct clinical guide to contact lens fitting and patient management, this book is all that is required. The succinct style, primarily in point form, makes it a genuine chair-side reference; that is, relevant, practical advice can be retrieved rapidly without having to wade through detailed background theory. Not that background theory is unimportant; it is vital and can be found elsewhere, but has been put aside in this book in the interests of clarity and immediacy.

The Contact Lens Manual: A Practical Fitting Guide is just that. This book will surely become a compulsory text for all students of optometry and ophthalmology, and will be a valuable chairside reference for the majority of practitioners who occasionally fit contact lenses and sometimes seek a little extra reassurance or assistance.

Andrew Gasson and Judith Morris are to be congratulated for producing this valuable and unique contribution to the contact lens literature. The publishers – Butterworth-Heinemann – also deserve recognition for their continuing commitment to producing quality optometric titles; *The Contact Lens Manual* is one volume of which they may be particularly proud.

Nathan Efron, PhD
Professor of Clinical Optometry
University of Manchester Institute of Science and Technology
United Kingdom

Preface

The Manual is designed as an essentially practical guide to all aspects of contact lens fitting. It follows the authors' own approach to patient management, initial assessment and lens selection as well as giving detailed fitting procedures for both basic and complex lenses. Significant space is allocated to aftercare as this is considered an inextricably linked continuation of fitting, whereas theoretical aspects have been kept deliberately concise, supplemented by detailed references and suggestions for further reading.

The introductory chapters and basic fitting are directed mainly at the student or practitioner without recent experience. *The Manual*, however, also covers advanced fitting techniques for the more experienced and the specialist sections on therapeutic lenses and the management of children requiring contact lenses should be of interest both to hospital fitters and to those who encounter the occasional medical case.

Terminology is based on the relatively new British and International Standards. The most common lens types are referred to as either 'hard' or 'soft'. The term 'hard' has been used throughout to indicate specifically modern materials which have been described elsewhere as 'gas-permeable'. PMMA is now considered a little-fitted sub-group.

Inevitably, it is impossible to include details of every lens or solution currently available and the authors have been forced to select representative examples. Mention of a particular product is not intended as an endorsement and any omission, however obvious, should not be construed as an implied criticism.

Finally, the authors would like to acknowledge all of the contact lens companies which have kindly made available detailed information concerning their products; the ACLM for the use of their materials classification system; Allergan-Hydron, Bausch and Lomb and Igel International for their permission to reproduce tables and illustrations; Tony Hough of Microturn for his assistance in producing the tear lens thickness diagrams; Ken Pullum for providing the basis of the section on scleral lenses and for his diagrams; and to the publishers for their constant help and encouragement.

APG
JAM

Chapter 1

Background

1.1 Applied anatomy

1.1.1 The cornea

Corneal tissue is transparent and avascular, consisting of three layers and two membranes. It protects the interior ocular structures and contributes 70% of the refractive power of the eye. It has the following average dimensions:

Radius of front surface 7.86 mm
Horizontal diameter 11.8 mm
Centre thickness 0.52 mm
Peripheral thickness 1.00 mm

Epithelium

Provides a layer of protective cells. It is enhanced by microvilli, which are prominent irregularities increasing the surface area and providing a roughened surface to assist the adherence of the precorneal tear film.

Very minor corneal insult is covered in about 3 hours by neighbouring cells. Larger areas of damage are covered by the migration of cells from all layers of the surrounding epithelium. Lesions close to the limbus show conjunctival cells taking part in the cell migration.

Practical advice

Newly regenerated epithelium is very susceptible to damage. Lens wear should be suspended for a few days following any significant degree of corneal trauma such as overwear or severe abrasion.

Bowman's membrane

The relatively tough anterior limiting layer of the cornea. It consists of a very fine non-orientated fibrillar meshwork. If Bowman's membrane is damaged, fibrous scar tissue is laid down, resulting in a permanent opacity.

Stroma

An avascular, regular structure which ensures both the mechanical strength and optical transparency of the cornea. Approximately 78% water, it represents about 90% of the corneal thickness.

Descemet's membrane

The posterior limiting layer of the cornea. It is the basement layer of the endothelium and is elastic in nature.

Endothelium

A single layer of cells in direct contact with the aqueous humour. Its pump mechanism maintains the cornea's fluid balance which is in turn responsible for transparency. No mitosis occurs, but enlargement and spreading of existing cells take place. Irregularity in the size of endothelial cells is termed *polymegathism*.

Corneal sensitivity

Innervation is by 70–80 sensory nerves entering the epithelium and usually losing their myelin sheaths within 0.5 mm of the limbus. The sensitivity of the cornea is greatest centrally and in the horizontal medium. It reduces towards the vertical and is least at the periphery. Conjunctival sensitivity increases from a minimum at the limbus towards a maximum at the fornix and lid margins.

Sensitivity reduces with age and with contact lens wear. It varies in women during the menstrual cycle and there is also a diurnal variation, with greatest sensitivity in the evening.

1.1.2 The conjunctiva

A mucous membrane, continuous with the corneal epithelium. It is divided into a bulbar portion which covers the anterior sclera and a palpebral portion which lines the tarsal plate of the eyelids. The conjunctival glands or goblet cells secrete the mucoproteins found in the tears.

1.1.3 The eyelids

The orbicularis oculi muscle makes up almost one-third of the eyelid thickness. Behind lies the tarsal plate which consists of dense fibrous tissue. The openings to the sebaceous meibomian glands lie in a single row along the lid margin. There are about 25 in the upper lid and 20 in the lower and they are best observed by eversion.

Practical advice

- Several contact lens problems relate to the eyelids so that lid eversion and thorough examination are essential prior to fitting.
- Meibomian gland dysfunction and blockage can contribute to dry eye symptoms.
- Infection of meibomian glands causes styes or cysts.
- The average blink rate is about once every 5 seconds.

1.1.4 The tear film

Functions

- Maintains a smooth optical surface over the cornea.
- Keeps the surface of the cornea moist.
- Acts as a lubricant for eyes and lids on blinking.
- Provides bacteriocidal action to protect corneal epithelium.
- Removes foreign bodies.

Composition

- An outermost oily, lipid layer secreted by the meibomium glands. Helps prevent evaporation.
- A central aqueous phase produced by the lacrimal gland and accessory glands of Krause and Wolfring.
- A mucoid layer, covering the epithelium, secreted by the conjunctival goblet cells.

The tear film is approximately 0.7 μm in thickness and about 90% of its volume is contained in the tear prism along the lid margin. The preocular tear film is adversely affected by the presence of a contact lens (*see* Section 3.6).

1.2 Applied physiology

A contact lens effectively occludes the cornea from its normal environment of oxygen, tears and ocular secretions. The effect depends upon lens thickness, size, method of fitting and material.

Corneal metabolism

Constant metabolic activity in the cornea maintains transparency, temperature, cell reproduction and the transport of tissue materials. The main nutrients needed for these functions are glucose, amino acids and oxygen. Glucose and amino acids are provided by the aqueous humour, whereas oxygen is mainly derived from the tears.

Each layer of the cornea consumes oxygen at a particular rate. Oxygen enters the cornea from both surfaces so that there is minimum tension in the stroma. *Oxygen tension* is the driving force that moves oxygen into the cornea. At sea level, it is 155 mm Hg for the open eye. Oxygen is supplied to the closed eye by the palpebral conjunctiva, where the tension is about 55 mm Hg [1].

Corneal swelling as a result of anoxia can be explained by biochemical theory [1]. In simple terms, there is not enough oxygen available to convert the glucose by means of glycolysis into sufficient energy and allow the waste product, lactic acid, to diffuse quickly out of the tissue. Less energy is therefore available for cellular activity, more lactic acid is produced and this builds up in the stroma. Sufficient osmotic pressure is created to allow water to be drawn into the stroma faster than the endothelial pump can remove it, and so corneal swelling occurs.

Corneal temperature

The normal corneal temperature of 33–36°C may alter during contact lens wear. The effect becomes more significant under closed eye conditions. The change in temperature may be only

3°C, but the rate of metabolic activity is so dependent on ambient temperature that the fine balance between available oxygen and corneal demands under the closed lid may be stressed by such a small temperature change.

Tear osmolarity

Corneal thickness is also affected by the osmolarity of the tears. In the normal, open eye the salt content of the tear film is about 10% greater than that of freshly produced tears due to evaporation. When the eye is closed during sleep, it is bathed by fresh isotonic tears. The cornea responds to the less concentrated solution by drawing water into the stroma faster than it can be pumped out by the endothelium. Hence, on wakening, the cornea is found to have increased in thickness by about 5% [2]. Deswelling occurs rapidly during the first 2 hours the eyes are open.

Tissue fragility

Reduced oxygen supply to the corneal epithelium, for example with extended wear, causes a decrease in the level of metabolic activity, including the rate of cell mitosis. The thickness of the epithelium reduces as cell production rate and wastage reach a new equilibrium. Such thinning has been observed in long-term extended wear patients. In addition, cell life increases and those at the anterior surface of the epithelium may not retain normal functional resistance. As a result of these changes, the overall resistance of the epithelium is lowered and the risk of infection increased.

Corneal sensitivity

One of the first, important effects of hypoxia, of which the patient is unaware, is a drop in corneal sensitivity [3].

Closed eyelid conditions during sleep

The following changes are induced:

- Increase in temperature.
- Hypotonic shift in tear osmolarity as a result of increased evaporation.

- Slight acidic shift in tear pH as a result of retardation of carbon dioxide efflux from the cornea.
- Corneal oxygenation reduced from 155 mm Hg (open eye) to 55 mm Hg (closed eye).

1.3 Physical properties of materials

1.3.1 Oxygen permeability, oxygen transmissibility and equivalent oxygen percentage

OXYGEN PERMEABILITY

The oxygen permeability of a material is generally referred to as the Dk. The units of 10^{-11} cm^2/s ml O$_2$/ml × mm Hg (sometimes referred to as Fatt units) are often omitted for convenience. In this nomenclature, D is the diffusion coefficient – a measure of how fast dissolved molecules of oxygen move within the material – and k is a constant representing the solubility coefficient or the number of oxygen molecules dissolved in the material.

The Dk value is a physical property of a contact lens material and describes its intrinsic ability to transport oxygen. It is defined as 'the rate of oxygen flow under specified conditions through unit area of contact lens material of unit thickness when subjected to unit pressure differences' [4]. It is not a function of the shape or thickness of the material sample, but varies with temperature. The higher the temperature, the greater the Dk [5].

OXYGEN TRANSMISSIBILITY

Oxygen transmissibility is referred to as Dk/t, with units of 10^{-9} cm/s ml O$_2$/ml × mm Hg. Here, t is the thickness of the lens or sample of material, and D and k are as defined above.

The Dk/t for a particular lens under specified conditions defines the ability of the lens to allow oxygen to move from anterior to posterior surface. The value of t is generally an average lens thickness for powers between ±3.00 dioptres (D). Outside of this range it is necessary to apply a nomogram [6]. Oxygen transmissibility is not a physical property of a contact lens material, but is a specific characteristic related to the sample thickness.

Surface effects

High Dk materials do not always give the oxygen performance on the eye that would be expected from laboratory results. The corneal swelling is equivalent to that of a lens with a *Dk* only 55% of the measured value [7]. This barrier effect is due to an intermediate water layer used in measurement. There is also an edge effect due to oxygen flow around the sample periphery [8].

Practical advice

Consistently reliable comparisons of various materials can be made only by the same person using the same instrument under identical conditions. Care is therefore required in comparing *Dk* measurements from different sources [9].

EQUIVALENT OXYGEN PERCENTAGE (EOP)

The equivalent oxygen percentage (EOP) refers to the level of oxygen at the surface of the cornea under a contact lens. For the uncovered cornea exposed to the atmosphere, the amount of oxygen available is 20.9%. With the eye closed the cornea receives 8%, whereas to avoid oedema the EOP should be over 10% [10] (*Dk/t* = 24.1), and for no overnight swelling it needs to be as high as 18% (*Dk/t* = 87). An EOP profile (Figure 1.1)

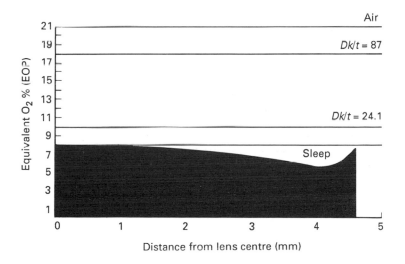

Figure 1.1 Equivalent oxygen percentage profile

for a lens of known material and thickness shows whether it can provide enough oxygen to avoid corneal oedema.

1.3.2 Water content and water uptake

The water content is the amount of fluid taken up by a lens material as a percentage of the whole under specified conditions:

Water content (%) =

$$\frac{\text{Wt of fully hydrated lens} - \text{Wt of fully dehydrated lens}}{\text{Wt of fully hydrated lens}} \times 100$$

Water uptake (%) =

$$\frac{\text{Wt of fully hydrated lens} - \text{Wt of fully dehydrated lens}}{\text{Wt of fully dehydrated lens}} \times 100$$

Water is lost by evaporation when a hydrogel lens is worn on the eye. This is in part caused by a rise in temperature and is accompanied by a tightening of the fit (*see* Section 17.3).

1.3.3 Wettability

Wettability is the ability of a drop of liquid to adhere to a solid surface. The lower the cohesive forces within a liquid, the greater the attraction between the fluid and surface. Thus, superior wettability enhances the spread of liquid over a surface.

Contact angle is a measure of the hydrophilicity of a surface. The contact angle may be measured in a variety of ways:

- Sessile drop method: measures the tangent to a drop of liquid placed on a sample surface (Figure 1.2).

- Captive bubble method: measures the tangent to an air bubble formed on the surface of an immersed sample.

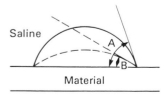

Saline

Material

Figure 1.2 Sessile drop method (A, advancing angle; B, receding angle)

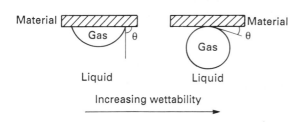

Increasing wettability

Figure 1.3 Captive bubble method

- Wilhelmy balance method. A sample is immersed or withdrawn vertically from a liquid [11].
- Direct meniscus method [11].

Both the advancing and receding angles are measured. These are formed when liquid is added to or removed from the controlled liquid drop used for measurement (Figure 1.2).

The higher the contact angle, the more wettable the surface. Typical values are given in Table 1.1, which demonstrates the great inconsistency between different methods. Comparisons can therefore only be made when the same method has been employed.

Table 1.1 Wetting angles

Material	Captive bubble*	Captive bubble†	Sessile†	Wilhelmy† Adv.	Wilhelmy† Rec.	Direct‡ Adv.	Direct‡ Rec.
PMMA	–	59.3	67.3	76.2	34.0	20	11
CAB	20	–	–	–	–	–	–
Boston II	21.5	36.5	82.7	74.0	27.4	46	14
Paraperm O₂	23.1	44.4	83.3	77.4	30.6	–	
Polycon II	15	–	–	–	–	–	–
	receding	–	–	–	–	–	–
Boston Equalens	30	–	–	–	–	–	–
Fluoromethacrylate (Quantum)	24	–	–	–	–	–	–

*From manufacturers' details.
†After Sarver *et al.* [12].
‡After Madigan, Holden and Fong [13].

PMMA, polymethyl methacrylate; CAB, cellulose acetate butyrate.

1.4 Methods of manufacture

The current trend is for soft lenses to be made cheaper and more reproducible by means of mass production, since the raw materials are relatively inexpensive. With hard lenses, however, the emphasis is on careful, stress-free manufacture, because the raw materials are costly and the laboratory is concerned to avoid waste.

1.4.1 Hard lens manufacture

- Conventional lathes to cut the back and front lens surfaces from buttons.
- Computer numerically controlled (CNC) lathes. Four types are available with different types of automation, so that both spherical and aspheric surfaces can be cut [14].

Polishing

The time and speed of polishing, together with the wetness and composition of the polish, are all very important. Frictional heating and over-polishing of the lens surface cause poor lens wettability.

1.4.2 Soft lens manufacture

- Lathing as with hard lenses, using buttons cut from rods. The finished lens is then hydrated.
- Spin casting, in which polymerization of the monomer and solvent takes place in open, spinning moulds (*see* Section 18).
- Cast moulding, which uses closed, disposable moulds with two components. Polymerization is by means of heat. The two methods are dry moulding, where the lens is moulded in the dry state and the edges finished by buffing; and wet moulding, in which the material is already hydrated (e.g. for disposable lenses).

References

1. Fatt, I. (1978) *Physiology of the Eye: An Introduction to the Vegetative Functions*, Butterworths, Boston
2. Mandell, R. and Fatt, I. (1965) Thinning of the human cornea on awakening. *Nature*, **208**, 292

3. Millodot, M. and O'Leary, D.J. (1980) Effect of oxygen deprivation on corneal sensitivity. *Acta Ophthalmologica*, **58**, 434
4. Fatt, I. and St. Helen, R. (1971) Oxygen tension under an oxygen permeable contact lens. *American Journal of Optometry*, **48**, 545
5. Morris, J.A. (1985) An overview of the hard gas permeable oxygen race. *Optometry Today*, **25**, 168–172
6. Brennan, N.A. (1984) Average thickness of a hydrogel lens for gas transmissibility calculations. *American Journal of Optometry*, **61**, 627
7. Brennan, N., Efron, N. and Holden, B.A. (1986) Further developments in the RGP *Dk* controversy. *International Eyecare*, **2**, 508–509
8. Fatt, I. (1986) Now do we need 'effective permeability'? *Contax*, July, 6–23
9. Holden, B.A., Newton-Howes, J., Winterton, L., Fatt, I., Hamano, H. and La Hood, D. *et al.* (1990) The *Dk* project: an interlaboratory comparison of *Dk/L* measurements. *Optometry and Vision Science*, **67**, 476–481
10. Holden, B.A. and Hertz, G.W. (1984) Critical oxygen levels to avoid corneal oedema for daily and extended wear contact lenses. *Investigative Ophthalmology and Visual Science*, **25**, 1161–1167
11. Pearson, R.M. (1987) Rigid gas permeable wettability and maintenance. *Contax*, Sept., 8–16
12. Sarver, M., Bowman, L., Bauman, E., Dimartino, R. and Umeda, W. (1984) Wettability of some gas permeable hard contact lenses. *International Contact Lens Clinic*, **11**, 479–490
13. Madigan, M., Holden, B.A. and Fong, D. (1986) A new method for wetting angle measurement. *International Eyecare*, **2**, 45–48
14. Hough, A. (1989) Contact lens production machinery. *Optician*, **197**(5205), 13–27

Chapter 2

Instrumentation

2.1 Slit lamp

The slit lamp provides the best method of observing ocular tissue in section under high magnification.

2.1.1 Instrument controls and focus

Instrument controls allow for variation in height, lateral movement and focusing. The illumination and observation systems are focused at a common point unless they are uncoupled to allow independent movement.

The optical system contains an *objective*, typically with ×3 to ×3.5 magnification, and an *eyepiece* with variable or interchangeable power. The normal range of total magnification gives ×6, ×10, ×16, ×25 and ×40.

Focus is achieved by rotating the slit beam about its fulcrum [1] (Figure 2.1).

● If the illuminated area moves with the direction of the arm, the projected slit is in front of the focus position.

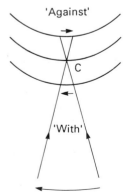

Figure 2.1 Focusing the slit beam (C, focus point)

- If the illuminated area moves against the direction of the arm, the projected slit is beyond the focus position.
- If the illuminated area remains stationary as the arm moves, the slit is exactly in focus.

2.1.2 Methods of illumination

DIRECT METHODS

The slit beam and microscope are focused at the same point to give:

- Diffuse illumination.
- Direct focal illumination.
- Indirect illumination.
- Specular reflection.
- Sclerotic scatter.

INDIRECT METHODS

The beam and microscope are uncoupled so that they are no longer focused at the same point to give:

- Indirect proper illumination.
- Sclerotic scatter.
- Retro-illumination.

2.1.3 Recommended slit lamp routine

- The instrument height is set for a half-way point in its travel range. The eyepieces are adjusted for the observer's prescription and pupillary distance (PD).
- A drop of fluorescein is instilled into each eye.
- The patient is made comfortable in relation to the height of headrest and instrument table.
- The patient closes the eyes and a slit beam is focused onto the eyelids. The beam is moved to the outer canthus without moving the instrument out of its range of focus, and the patient asked to open eyes.
- Diffuse illumination is used for a general look at the ocular tissues under low magnification.
- In a darkened room, the cornea is examined with sclerotic

scatter using either the microscope or the unaided eye for signs of opacities or oedema.

- Starting at the temporal limbus, the corneal tissue is scanned using direct focal illumination and a parallelepiped at least 2 mm wide. The slit beam is set between 40° and 60° to the temporal side of the centrally placed microscope. Magnification should be about ×20. From the corneal apex to the nasal limbus the illumination system can be swung to the nasal side of the microscope.

- The beam is reduced to an optic section and the cornea examined in the same manner, localizing any abnormality discovered with the wide beam.

- The patient looks up and down, to take in the superior and inferior limbal areas.

- The direct slit beam is oscillated as the cornea is traversed. Any abnormality changes the scattering of light in the tissues and aids identification. The whole field of view contained by the beam and its surrounds is continuously observed with a combination of direct and indirect illumination.

- As the direct beam is moved across the cornea, specular reflection of the tear film occurs. Examination of this bright area, looking for any debris or oiliness, gives a qualitative assessment of the tear film. Changing focus to the rear of the beam section brings an area of endothelium into view (Figure 2.2). A general idea of endothelial regularity is obtained, rather than specific cell details. Each zone appears double, as the reflected light using this method enters only one eyepiece at a time.

N.B. The endothelium looks like a patch of beaten gold to the side of the much brighter specular zone.

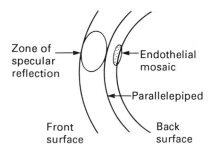

Zone of specular reflection

Endothelial mosaic

Parallelepiped

Front surface

Back surface

Figure 2.2 Specular reflection showing the endothelium

- The slit lamp is uncoupled to examine the cornea by means of retro-illumination. Direct, marginal and indirect retro-illumination ascertain whether any abnormality is more or less dense than the surrounding tissue. This is revealed by the way the light converges or diverges around the abnormality, and aids in its identification [2].
- Both the cornea and conjunctiva are then examined for evidence of epithelial staining using a broad scanning beam and the cobalt blue filter. A yellow filter (Kodak Wratten 12) in the observation system gives enhanced contrast and assists identification. Other stains used are rose bengal and less commonly alcian blue.

Practical advice

Correct use of the slit lamp requires the co-ordinated use of both hands – one to control the joystick and the other the slit beam.

2.2 Keratometer (ophthalmometer)

Keratometers measure the curvature of the central cornea over an area of approximately 3–6 mm to determine:

- The radii of curvature.
- The directions of the principal meridians.
- The degree of corneal astigmatism.
- The presence of any corneal distortion.

Practical advice

The same cornea measured with more than one instrument can result in a variety of readings because different keratometers employ:

- Different mire separations, so that the area of cornea used for reflection varies.
- Different refractive indices for calibration, so that the same radius could give a variety of surface powers.

2.2.1 Types of keratometer

There are two types of instrument, depending on the system of doubling employed to measure the separation of the mire images. Doubling helps in taking the reading, since rapid eye movements would otherwise make the measurement extremely difficult.

Variable doubling

The mires have a fixed separation. The separation of the mire images is found by varying the doubling power. The Bausch and Lomb keratometer has two variable doubling devices and two sets of fixed mires (Figure 2.3). Both principal meridians can

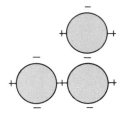

Figure 2.3 Bausch and Lomb mires

therefore be measured simultaneously, and it is called a 'one position' instrument.

Fixed doubling

The doubling is fixed for a particular separation of the mire images. It is only by altering the separation of the mires themselves that a reading can be taken. These keratometers are called 'two position' instruments and are based on the Javal–Shiötz design (Figure 2.4).

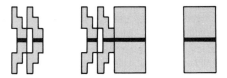

Figure 2.4 Javal-Schiötz mires

2.2.2 Focusing the eyepiece

Most keratometers have a graticule incorporated in the eyepiece. This should be focused prior to taking a reading to prevent accommodation giving an inaccurate result.

2.2.3 Taking a measurement

The patient should be comfortably seated, with the forehead positioned firmly against the headrest. Fixation should be accurate, with the other eye occluded. To help line up the optical system and locate the patient's cornea use:

- the sights attached to the instrument;
- the light from a pen torch directed through the eyepiece, looking for the corneal reflection.

The instrument is positioned initially at a greater distance from the cornea than necessary and slowly moved forward until the mire images come into view and are sharply focused. There should be four images, two of each mire either side of the centre. The middle pair are brought together until lined up in the correct position to take a reading (Figure 2.4).

Similar images need to be superimposed (Figure 2.5), whereas dissimilar mires are required to touch (Figure 2.4). In each case,

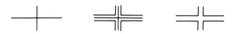

Figure 2.5 Superimposed images – Zeiss (Oberkochen) mires

the instrument is rotated to orientate with the first principal meridian. The measurement is recorded and the second principal meridian found by rotating the instrument through 90°.

Practical advice

- The principal meridians are not at 90° with an irregular cornea.
- Instruments usually show the corneal radius in both millimetres and dioptres.
- The power and radius scales have their maximum and minimum values at opposite ends.
- The axis of the meridian is usually obtained from an external protractor scale.
- Keratometry readings are expressed as *along* a particular meridian.
- Patients fitted in the USA generally have their keratometry and lenses specified in dioptres.

2.2.4 Extending the range

Radii steeper than the range of the instrument (e.g. keratoconus) can be obtained by placing a +1.25 D trial lens in front of the keratometer objective. At the flatter end, the range can be similarly extended with a −1.00 D lens. Prior calibration is necessary using steel balls of known radius [3].

Practical advice

For keratoconus, the Javal–Schiötz instrument is particularly useful, because the range at the steep end extends as far as 5.50 mm.

2.2.5 Topographical keratometer

The keratometer can also be used to explore the paracentral and peripheral areas of the cornea by means of a graduated fixation attachment [4].

2.3 Other instruments

Burton lamp

The Burton lamp uses ultraviolet light at a safe wavelength of about 400 nm. The lamp is also referred to as a 'blue light' or 'black light' and is used in conjunction with fluorescein (*see* Section 9.2.1).

Most Burton lamps are combined with a low power magnifier, large enough to permit binocular viewing. Many models combine white light tubes and some incorporate a yellow filter to intensify the fluorescence.

Placido disc

The Placido disc is a flat circular disc with alternate black and white concentric rings. The width and separation of the rings increase towards the periphery and are designed so that the reflections appear the same width when reflected from an average cornea. It gives a qualitative assessment of the regularity of the cornea itself. The eye is viewed through a convex lens in the centre of the disc.

Klein keratoscope

The Klein keratoscope is an internally illuminated version of the Placido disc.

Computer analysis

The photoelectric keratoscope (PEK) produced a photographic record of corneal topography. It explored the paracentral and peripheral areas of the cornea. The information could be used to provide a computer-designed contact lens (e.g. the Wesley–Jessen system). More modern computer analysis (e.g. Eyesys) can give a much more detailed assessment of overall corneal topography.

References

1. Stone, J. (1979) The slit lamp biomicroscope in ophthalmic practice. *Ophthalmic Optician*, **19**, 439–454
2. Phelps Brown, N. (1989) Mini pathology of the eye. *Optician*, **197**(5200), 22–29
3. Sampson, W.G. and Soper, J.W. (1970) Keratometry. In *Corneal Contact Lenses*, 2nd edn, L.J. Girard (ed.), Mosby, St. Louis
4. Wilms, K.H. and Rabbetts, R.B. (1977) Practical concepts of corneal topometry. *Optician*, **174**(4502), 7–13

Chapter 3

Preliminary considerations and examination

3.1 Discussion with the patient

It is important to discuss the various aspects of contact lenses at the first examination and assess potential suitability in relation to patient expectations, spectacle refraction, 'K' readings and slit lamp examination. The discussion, however, should cover many other related aspects of lens wear and fitting:

- General health, including allergies, hay fever and systemic drugs.
- Ocular health, previous infections or surgery.
- Vision, nature of Rx, amblyopia.
- Previous contact lens history, success or failure.
- Reasons for contact lens wear.
- Types of lens currently available.
- Preconceived ideas and misconceptions.
- Outline of fitting procedures.
- What is required of the patient in terms of aftercare examinations, hygiene and proper use of solutions.
- Fees for both initial fitting and future aftercare.

3.2 Indications and contraindications

3.2.1 Advantages and disadvantages compared with spectacles

ADVANTAGES

- Wider field of view.
- Better for refractive anisometropia.
- Retinal image size almost normal with refractive ametropia (e.g. with aphakia, high minus).

- No unwanted prismatic effects with eye movements.
- Less convergence required by hyperopes for near vision.
- Avoid surface reflections.
- Minimal oblique or other aberrations.
- Cosmetically superior.
- More practical for sports.
- Avoid weather problems (rain, snow, fogging-up).
- Provide good acuity for irregular corneas (keratoconus, scarring).
- Therapeutic uses.
- Vocational uses.

DISADVANTAGES

- Time required for fitting and adaptation.
- Handling skills required by patient.
- Lens disinfection necessary.
- Wearing time may be limited.
- Range of useful tints limited.
- Only limited vertical prism possible for binocular problems.
- Greater convergence required by myopes for near vision.
- Lenses can be lost or broken.
- Problems with foreign bodies.
- Peripheral flare (especially at night).
- Deteriorate with use and age.
- Retinal image size disparity in axial anisometropia.
- Maintenance costs.
- Greater overall expense.

3.2.2 Indications and contraindications

INDICATIONS

There are many patients for whom contact lenses are not merely a matter of cosmetic choice, but the best means of providing a satisfactory visual correction.

Visual

- Anisometropia.
- High myopia.
- Aphakia.
- Irregular corneas, scarring, keratoconus, grafts.

Occupational

- Theatre and film performers.
- Armed forces.
- Professional sports.

Cosmetic

- To avoid spectacles.
- Change eye colour.
- Prosthetic lenses or shells.

Medical

- Therapeutic.
- Bandage.

Psychological

- Where the patient cannot accept wearing spectacles.

Other

- Sports.
- Physical inability to wear spectacles (e.g. allergy to frame materials, nasal problems).

CONTRAINDICATIONS

There are a great many factors which may be considered as contraindications. Few of them are absolute, but all must be carefully assessed prior to fitting.

Visual

- Low refractive errors (e.g. +1.00/−0.75, −0.25/−0.50).
- Correction required only for near vision.
- Acuity with lenses may be worse than with spectacles.
- Prism required horizontally or >3 vertically.

Occupational

- Where legal constraints apply.

Cosmetic

- Where spectacles are better with a large-angle squint.
- Where spectacles hide facial disfigurement.

Medical

- Active infection or pathology.
- Recurrent corneal erosions.
- Severe sinus or catarrhal problems.
- Allergies.
- Vernal catarrh.
- Diabetes (fragile epithelium).
- Anatomical (e.g. misshapen lid).

Psychological

- Cannot accept the idea of a lens on the eye.
- Cannot tolerate any level of discomfort.
- Unable to cope with insertion and removal.
- Total perfectionist.

Sensitivity

- Cornea too sensitive.
- Lids or lid margins too sensitive.

Dryness

- Poor volume or quality of tears.

- Poor blinking.
- Dry environment.
- Drug-induced (e.g. antihistamine).
- Job-induced (e.g. VDUs).

Environment

- Dust.
- Fumes.
- Dryness (central heating, air conditioning, aeroplanes).
- Altitude (low EOP).

3.3 Advantages and disadvantages of lens types

The most common lens types are referred to as either 'hard' or 'soft'. **The term 'hard' has been used throughout to indicate specifically modern materials which have been described elsewhere as 'gas permeable'.** PMMA is now considered a little-fitted subgroup.

3.3.1 Hard lenses

ADVANTAGES

- Good visual acuity.
- Correct corneal astigmatism.
- Variety of complex designs available.
- Ease of maintenance.
- Few solutions allergies.
- Few deposits.
- High oxygen permeabilities (*Dk*s).
- Tear pump on blinking.
- Good long-term ocular response.
- Easy to check.
- Modifications possible.
- Lenses available in a range of tints.

DISADVANTAGES

- Initial discomfort.
- Precise fitting required.
- Foreign bodies.
- Risk of loss.
- Flare.
- 3 and 9 o'clock staining.
- Lens adhesion.
- Breakage and scratching.
- Instability of some materials.

3.3.2 PMMA lenses

ADVANTAGES

- Inertness of material.
- Stability of material.
- Reproducibility.
- Surface wettability.
- Quality of vision.
- Myopia control.
- Ease of manufacture.
- Ease of modification.
- Range of tints.
- Inexpensive.

DISADVANTAGES

- Slow adaptation.
- High incidence of oedema.
- Corneal distortion.
- Spectacle blur.
- Risk of overwear syndrome.
- Endothelial polymegathism.
- Severely reduced corneal sensitivity.

3.3.3 Soft lenses

ADVANTAGES

- Good initial comfort.
- Ease of adaptation.
- Natural facial expression and head posture.
- Long wearing times.
- Low incidence of oedema.
- Rare occurrence of overwear syndrome.
- Absence of spectacle blur.
- Maintenance of corneal sensitivity.
- Good for intermittent wear.
- Low incidence of photophobia and lacrimation.
- Low incidence of flare, even with large pupils.
- Few problems with foreign bodies.
- Low risk of loss.
- Good for sports.

DISADVANTAGES

- Astigmatism not corrected with spherical lenses.
- Variable vision.
- Near vision problems.
- Lens dehydration.
- Liable to damage.
- Deposits and lens ageing.
- Disinfection essential.
- Solutions allergies.
- Lens cleaning more difficult.
- Lens contamination.
- Limited life span.
- No modifications possible.
- Difficult to check.
- Corneal vascularization.
- Papillary conjunctivitis (PC).
- Expensive to maintain.

3.4 Visual considerations

CORNEAL AND RESIDUAL ASTIGMATISM

Two basic assumptions are made when assessing the potential success of patients with astigmatism:

(1) Total ocular astigmatism = corneal astigmatism + lenticular astigmatism.
(2) Most corneal astigmatism is transferred through a soft lens to its anterior surface.

Patients may therefore be divided into four groups at their initial examination by reference to spectacle correction and 'K' readings.

Spherical cornea with spherical refraction

Rx: −3.00 DS
'K': 7.85 mm along 180° (43.00 D)
     7.85 mm along 90° (43.00 D)

This is the ideal optical case for contact lens fitting. Vision should be equally good with either hard or soft lenses.

Spherical cornea with astigmatic refraction

Rx: −2.00/−1.75 × 90
'K': 7.85 mm along 180° (43.00 D)
     7.90 mm along 90° (42.75 D)

The astigmatism is almost entirely lenticular, so that the visual result is the same with either a hard or a soft lens. In either case, a front surface toric lens is required to correct the 1.50 D of residual astigmatism.

Toric cornea with astigmatic refraction

Rx: −2.00/−1.75 × 180
'K': 7.80 mm along 180° (43.25 D)
     7.50 mm along 90° (45.00 D)

All of the astigmatism is corneal. A spherical hard lens, which neutralizes 90% of corneal astigmatism, or a toric soft lens should therefore be fitted.

Toric cornea with spherical refraction

Rx: −3.00 D
'K': 7.80 mm along 180° (43.25 D)
     7.50 mm along 90° (45.00 D)

There is 1.75 D of with-the-rule corneal astigmatism together with an equivalent degree of against-the-rule lenticular astigmatism, giving a resultant spherical refraction. A hard lens form would neutralize the corneal but *not* the lenticular astigmatism. It would therefore leave a residual cylinder of −1.75 × 90. A soft lens should be used *because* it transfers all of the corneal astigmatism through to its front surface without optically neutralizing it.

General advice

Where there is an equal choice between fitting either a toric hard or toric soft, because of the much greater comfort it is generally better to fit a soft lens.

NEAR VISION

Near vision can often cause problems despite good distance acuity. There are several reasons [1], the main ones being:

● Altered accommodation/convergence ratio.

● Low myopes who previously did not wear spectacles.

● Early presbyopes requiring greater accommodation with lenses compared with spectacles. Conversely, hypermetropes are usually delighted with improved near vision.

INTERMEDIATE VISION

Intermediate visual tasks such as VDU operation or painting can also cause problems. Particular difficulties occur with reading music, especially in dim illumination.

CONTRAST SENSITIVITY AND 'QUALITY OF VISION'

Contact lenses of all types do not always give the absolute stability of vision achieved with spectacles. Variations may be due to either the lens or environmental factors. The 'quality of vision' is very much a subjective interpretation and does not necessarily correlate with Snellen acuity. This can be confirmed by marked differences in contrast sensitivity readings while visual acuity remains the same [2].

MONOCULAR PATIENTS

Particular care is necessary when fitting essentially monocular patients. They are much more disturbed by factors such as lens mobility, flare or unstable vision with toric and bifocal lenses.

Practical advice

- Stability of vision is often as important as acuity.
- Snellen acuity is not always a reliable guide to a patient's potential success. In some circumstances a good 6/9 may be more acceptable than a poor 6/6.
- Assess distance, near and intermediate vision separately in relation to work and visual requirements.
- Take particular care with monocular patients.

3.5 External eye examination

External examination prior to fitting is essential to allow the practitioner to:

- Confirm the normality of ocular tissues.
- Discover any condition which would preclude contact lens wear.
- Record for the future any other abnormality.
- Refer for medical treatment any active disease unrelated to contact lens considerations.

Most parts of the examination are carried out using the slit lamp (see Section 2.1.3), looking for any evidence of the following conditions.

Cornea and limbus

● Vascularization or neovascularization.
● Staining.
● Desiccation.
● Infiltrates or other signs of previous infection.
● Scarring or opacification.
● Other signs of injury.
● Central thinning.
● Peripheral thinning (dellen).
● Pterygium.

Bulbar conjunctiva

● Injection.
● Desiccation.
● Pinguecula.
● Other irregularity.

Lids

● Position and size of palpebral aperture.
● Lid tension.
● Irregularity of lid margins.
● Styes and cysts.
● Blepharitis.
● General condition of skin.
● Vesicles on lid margins.
● Patency of meibomian glands.
● Vernal conjunctivitis.
● Papillary conjunctivitis (PC).
● Concretions.
● Make-up on palpebral conjunctiva.

Blinking

● Frequency.
● Completeness.

Practical advice

- Lid eversion to examine the tarsal plate and papillary conjunctiva is an essential preliminary.
- Most patients find it rather unpleasant.
- Eversion also gives clues to sensitivity and to how patients will react to having their eyes manipulated.
- Where eversion proves very difficult, it is often possible to examine sufficient of the papillary conjunctiva by instructing the patient to hold the head as far back as possible and look down. The upper lid is gently pulled away from the globe and the light from a pen torch directed towards the upper fornix.

3.6 Assessment of tears

Assessment of tears is an important part of the preliminary examination in order to:

- Predict potential success.
- Eliminate likely failures.
- Discover marginally dry eyes which would be adversely affected by a contact lens.
- Decide on the most appropriate lens type.

There are several ways of assessing the tears. Each has its own limitations depending upon factors such as temperature, humidity and whether the method is invasive or non-invasive.

3.6.1 Assessment of the tear volume

Tear prism observation

The upper and lower tear prisms hold 90% of the tear volume, so that the height and width give a reasonable assessment of tear volume.

- Slit lamp observation either with or without fluorescein gives an overall view of the entire prism.
- The approximate height of the prism in a normal tear film is 0.2–0.4 mm at the centre and 0.1–0.2 mm at the periphery [3].
- Reduced height suggests reduced tear volume.

- Increased height could indicate poor drainage because of obstructed puncta or an excessive aqueous layer giving a watery tear film.
- The regularity of the prism along the length of the lid margins indicates the potential of the film to wet the eye consistently. This reduces with age.
- Frothing of the tears within the prism indicates lipid contamination, probably due to meibomium gland dysfunction.

Practical advice

- Measurement of the prism is largely an estimate based on experience.
- To gain this experience, routinely observe all patients to get used to the norm. Initially, aim to recognize an obviously defective prism of half normal height and subsequently refine observation to three-quarters of normal. The value in millimetres is less important than the departure from normal.
- Insertion of fluorescein destabilizes the tear film and can increase the height of the prism.

Schirmer test

This is a quantitative test of tear production which uses strips of Whatman No. 1 filter paper with notched ends 5 mm wide (Figure 3.1).

The notched end is folded twice to give better balance on the lower lid and placed against the bulbar conjunctiva near the

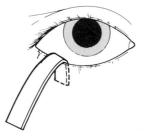

Figure 3.1 Schirmer tear production test

outer canthus. The eye looks up and in, to avoid contact with the cornea. The lower lid is released to retain the folded part in place. The remainder of the strip projects at right-angles from the lid.

The result is recorded either as the length of paper moistened in 5 min (normal = 15 mm) or the time taken to wet a length of 10 mm (normal = 3 min).

Practical advice

● The invasive nature of the strip causes reflex tearing.

● The results do not necessarily represent the patient's norm, but do indicate the presence or absence of reflex lacrimation.

● The result is quantitative and can be recorded for future comparison.

Phenol red thread

The test consists of a cotton, two-ply thread impregnated with phenol red (phenolsulphonphthalein). The thread is pH sensitive and changes from yellow to red as it is wetted by the tears [4]. The normal result gives 10–20 mm moistened in 15 s.

3.6.2 Tear film stability

Tear break-up time (BUT)

The tear break-up time (BUT) is the time in seconds for the break-up of the precorneal tear film in a non-blinking eye. It is a convenient and simple test to perform, but its invasive nature requires careful interpretation of the results.

A drop of fluorescein is instilled into the eye. The slit lamp with blue light is used to observe the patient after a few blinks have mixed the fluorescein completely into the tear film. The patient stares while a wide blue beam is focused onto the cornea. The time is recorded for the first break in the tear film, shown as a dark blue patch against the otherwise green background of fluorescein.

A normal result gives a BUT of 15 s or greater.

Practical advice

- If 15 s elapse with no break in the tear film, ask the patient to relax since the tear film is well within normal limits and the test can become uncomfortable after about 20 s.

- The position of the first break is often significant, especially if it corresponds to an area of staining or occurs at the lower limbus, since it suggests potential problems of desiccation.

- A supplementary test, possibly of even greater value, is to observe the relaxed patient blinking normally to determine whether the tear film breaks up between blinks or remains unbroken until the next blink.

- The use of fluorescein destabilizes the tear film and can give erroneous results.

- The temperature and humidity of the consulting room can affect the result.

- Only a large variation in results (5–10 s) is significant.

Other tests

- Non-invasive break-up time methods measure the stability of the tear film without any staining agent. They use either a specially designed cold diffuse light source [5] or a grid pattern to indicate the tear film pre-rupture phase time (TP-RPT) [6,7].

- Observing the bright zone of specular reflection with the slit lamp (*see* Section 2.1.3) allows debris in the tears to show up as dark spots which move on blinking.

- The first Purkinje image, seen with reduced slit lamp illumination, appears either plain or enhanced with coloured fringes. It gives a relative estimate of tear film thickness and can indicate contamination of the lipid layer. Coloured fringes alone are difficult to assess, but when found together with irregularity of the tear prism they strongly suggest a poor tear film.

3.7 Patient suitability for lens types

The majority of patients are now fitted with either hard or soft lenses. PMMA, scleral or other lens forms are needed only occasionally. It is often immediately obvious from the preliminary examination and discussion which type is likely to be more suitable. Many patients can be successful with either hard or soft lenses, but it is quite often necessary actually to use trial lenses of each type in order to evaluate lens performance on the eye.

3.7.1 Hard lenses

Hard lenses are the likely first choice in the following cases:

NEW PATIENTS

● Soft trial lenses give unsatisfactory vision.
● Significant corneal astigmatism is present (>1.00 D).
● Corneal irregularity is present.
● Dry eyes have been diagnosed.
● An extremely high Dk is required.
● VDUs are used full-time.
● Dry geographic or working environment.
● There is a history of hay fever, vernal conjunctivitis or PC prior to fitting.
● The appearance of the limbal vessels prior to fitting suggests that vascularization is a likely consequence with soft lenses.
● Patients are unlikely to manage soft lens disinfection.
● Handling difficulties are likely with soft lenses (e.g. low myopes with ultra-thin lenses; very small palpebral apertures).
● Lenses are likely to require future power modification.

REFITS OR PREVIOUS FAILURES

Where soft lenses have failed because of:

● Poor vision.
● Poor comfort.
● Dry eyes.
● Poor centration or fitting.
● Poor handling or repeated breakage.

- Corneal vascularization.
- PC.
- Repeated infections.
- Unacceptably short life span.
- Frequent deposits.
- Solutions allergies.
- Materials allergy.

3.7.2 Soft lenses

Soft lenses are the likely first choice in the following cases:

NEW PATIENTS

- Hard trial lenses give unsatisfactory comfort because the lids or cornea are obviously too sensitive.
- Hard trial lenses give poor centration.
- The *Rx* is spherical and hypermetropic.
- The *Rx* is spherical with astigmatic 'K' readings (*see* Section 3.4).
- The pupils are very large or decentred.
- Rapid adaptation is required.
- An irregular wearing schedule is expected.
- Older patients.
- There are awkward anatomical features likely to give poor hard lens positioning (e.g. low lower lid; proptosed eyes; decentred corneal apex).
- Dusty geographic or working environment.
- Patients need the security of a lens which it is almost impossible to dislodge from the eye (e.g. professional sports use).

REFITS OR PREVIOUS FAILURES

Where hard lenses have failed because of:

- Poor comfort.
- Poor vision.
- Flare and reflections.

- Poor centration.
- Oedema.
- Poor blinking.
- 3 and 9 o'clock staining or vascularization.
- Other persistent corneal staining.
- Persistent conjunctival injection.
- Poor handling or repeated loss.

References

1. Stone, J. (1967) Near vision difficulties in non-presbyopic corneal lens wearers. *Contact Lens Journal*, **1**, 14–16
2. Guillan, H., Lydon, D.P.M and Wilson, C. (1983) Variations in contrast Sensitivity function with spectacles and contact lenses. *Journal of the British Contact Lens Association*, **6**, 120–124
3. Osbourne, G., Zantos, S., Robboy, M., Medici, L. and Petrzala, L. (1989) Evaluation of tear meniscus heights on marginal dry eye soft lens wearers. *Investigative Ophthalmology and Visual Science*, **30** (suppl.), 501
4. Hamano, H. and Kaufman, H.E. (1987) *The Physiology of the Cornea and Contact Lens Applications*, Churchill Livingstone, New York
5. Guillon, J-P. (1986) Observing and photographing the pre corneal and pre lens tear film. *Contax*, Nov., 15–22
6. Mengher, L.S., Bron, A.J., Tonge, S.R. and Gilbert, D.J. (1985) A non-invasive instrument for clinical assessment of the pre-corneal tear film stability. *Current Eye Research*, **4**, 1–7
7. Hirji, N., Patel, S. and Callender, M. (1989) Human tear film pre-rupture phase time (TP-RPT) a non-invasive technique for evaluating the pre-corneal tear film using a novel keratometer mire. *Ophthalmic and Physiological Optics*, **9**, 139–142

Chapter 4

Consulting room procedures and equipment

Hygienic procedures within the consulting room are extremely important to avoid any risk of cross-infection between patients as well as between patient and practitioner [1].

4.1 Solutions and drugs

Water

Water may be used for rinsing hard lenses, and prior to their insertion with a suitable wetting solution. It should not be used with soft lenses because of potential problems of contamination [2] and the likelihood of hypotonic adhesion to the cornea.

Saline (0.9% sodium chloride BP)

Normal saline is extensively used in contact lens practice for a variety of applications:

● Ocular irrigation.
● Rinsing lenses prior to insertion.
● Rinsing and cleaning lenses after fitting.
● Heat disinfection of soft lenses and subsequent storage.
● Wet cells of instruments for soft lens verification.
● Wetting fluorescein strips.
● Rewetting soft lenses.

Practical advice
● For soft lenses, use unpreserved saline.
● For hard lenses, use either preserved or unpreserved saline. Avoid aerosols for insertion because of air bubbles trapped under the lens.

● Saline can no longer be prepared from salt tablets and purified water because of the risk of contamination.

Proprietary solutions

A range of proprietary wetting, soaking and cleaning solutions is required for both hard and soft lenses (*see* Chapter 25).

STAINING AGENTS

Fluorescein sodium BP

Used in 1% or 2% solution or, more usually, as impregnated paper strips which can be stored indefinitely if kept dry. Cross-infection is avoided by using a different strip for each patient and in some case for each eye.

Fluorescein is the main method of checking hard lens fitting. It makes the tear pattern visible either by means of ultraviolet fluorescence with a Burton lamp or with the cobalt filter of the slit lamp. Fluorescein is almost entirely washed out of the eye within the hour, but a saline rinse is recommended before soft lens reinsertion to avoid any risk of discolouration. It is an important diagnostic aid because it stains damaged living corneal tissue green and the conjunctiva yellow. Observation with the slit lamp is made easier if a yellow Wratten 12 filter is used.

High molecular weight fluorescein (e.g. Fluoresoft or Fluorexon)

The molecular weight is sufficiently great to prevent immediate penetration into soft lens materials. The degree of fluorescence is much less than with standard fluorescein and the technique is of limited value.

Rose bengal 1%

Stains devitalized epithelial cells of the cornea and conjunctiva bright red. Indicates abnormal ocular conditions or skin disease. Causes mild discomfort on insertion and takes several hours to absorb. Also stains mucus.

Alcian blue

Stains mucus blue, but is not used in contact lens practice as traces remain in the eye for too long.

TOPICAL ANAESTHETICS

Benoxinate 0.4%; amethocaine 0.5% and 1.0%

Primarily used prior to taking eye impressions. Anaesthetics tend to retard healing of the corneal epithelium and in cases of trauma and overwear are used only in the presence of extreme pain.

ANTIMICROBIAL AGENTS

Chloramphenicol BP 0.5% (chloromycetin)

A broad-spectrum antibiotic normally used in emergency as a prophylactic, ophthalmic anti-infective.

Brolene (0.1% propamidine isethionate)

Antibiotic with some efficacy against acanthamoeba [3].

OTHER DRUGS

Sodium cromoglycate 2% (Opticrom)

An anti-allergic, antihistaminic preparation to reduce inflammation and mucus secretion. Used generally for a period of 28 days in the treatment of PC to stop irritation, mucus production and growth of papillae. Generally effective in reducing symptoms but not always the size of papillae.

Adrenaline 0.1%

A conjunctival decongestant, often used after taking eye impressions.

Sodium bicarbonate 2%

Used to fill sealed scleral lenses on insertion and for ocular irrigation.

4.2 Trial lens disinfection

HARD AND PMMA LENSES

After removal from the eye, hard lenses should be carefully cleaned and stored in a proprietary soaking solution. Low-powered PMMA lenses can be stored dry, but require careful rewetting before insertion.

Practical advice

Avoid very viscous solutions for storage. Lenses left for any length of time can be extremely difficult to remove from the vial.

SOFT LENSES

It is essential that soft lenses are disinfected before use with another patient. A 'quarantine' area can be set aside for this purpose and several disinfection methods are possible after surfactant cleaning:

● Heat. autoclaving in 0.9% saline is arguably the safest method, but high temperature can adversely affect the life span of some high water content lenses.

● Preserved solutions are the most convenient method, but 4–6 h are required before lenses can be re-used, and some patients are sensitive to the preservatives.

● Most hydrogen peroxide systems require less times, but the procedures are complicated for routine trial lens storage.

● Chlorine tablets represent a convenient method in practice, but some patients experience stinging with high water content lenses stored in vials too small to allow the correct concentration.

4.3 Other procedures

4.3.1 Professional cleaning and rejuvenation

HARD AND PMMA LENSES

A modification unit is used to repolish hard lenses, recondition the lens surface and make other adjustments (*see* Section 28.6).

SOFT LENSES

Magnetic stirrers incorporating a hotplate efficiently clean most soft lenses using oxidizing chemicals such as Liprofin (*see* Section 25.4.5).

Ultrasonic devices are claimed to have a cleaning and disinfecting action with both soft and hard lenses.

4.3.2 Lens verification

The instruments for hard and soft lens verification are covered respectively in Sections 11.3 and 19.3.

Practical advice

- Keep a projection magnifier in the consulting room both for lens checking and for demonstrating lens condition to the patient.
- Regularly clean and disinfect wet cells filled with saline, since they are a potential source of contamination. Hydrogen peroxide is generally the best method, but for any particular instrument seek the manufacturer's advice to ensure there is no risk of damage.

4.3.3 Ancillary items

The following ancillary items are frequently required during fitting:

- Soft-ended tweezers, a lens lift or glass rod for removing soft lenses from their vials.
- A glass rod or muscle hook is also useful for removing a dislodged lens from the upper fornix.
- Suction holders for use with hard lenses.
- Clean lens mailers for temporary storage when lenses are removed from the eye during examination.
- Glass vials or lens cases for storage when lenses are retained for professional cleaning.
- A crimping device for resealing pharmaceutical lens vials.
- Small self-adhesive labels for identifying lenses temporarily stored in unmarked bottles.
- Miscellaneous items, including facial rule, grease pencil, pupil gauge and pen torch.

4.4 Insertion and removal by the practitioner

Practical advice

- Ensure the patient is as relaxed as possible.
- Avoid the patient actually seeing the lens approach.
- Ensure both eyes remain open because of Bell's phenomenon.
- Keep the eyes still and slightly depressed by using a fixation target below eye level.
- The head and neck should lean firmly against a carefully positioned headrest.
- Stand at the side of the patient.
- Establish whether lids are tight or loose, as this may influence the choice of method.

4.4.1 Hard and PMMA lenses

INSERTION

- The patient looks with both eyes either at a fixation target just below the horizontal or down at the floor.
- The upper lid is retracted.
- The lens is placed onto the cornea from above using either the forefinger or a suction holder.

With very tight-lidded patients and where fixation cannot be controlled:

- The patient looks to the extreme nasal position.
- The lens is placed onto the temporal sclera and gently slid across to the cornea.

Once the lens is in position, the patient is advised not to look up, but to half close the eyes and look down to minimize lid sensation.

REMOVAL

- The head is leaned firmly back into the headrest.
- The patient fixates straight ahead.

- The lens is ejected with pressure applied either at the top and bottom lid margins or at the outer canthus.
- Alternatively, the lens is removed from the cornea with a moistened suction holder.

4.4.2 Soft lenses

INSERTION

Soft lenses may be inserted either onto the temporal sclera and slid across or in the same way as hard lenses and placed directly onto the cornea.

Practical advice

- If placed on the cornea with an air bubble, lenses are unstable at the moment of insertion and can be expelled by an involuntary blink.
- Most lenses (except ultra-thin) self-centre onto the cornea.
- Place ultra-thin lenses directly onto the cornea.
- In difficult cases, allow the lens to dry on the finger for 15–30 s to prevent it from turning inside out and make it easier for the tear film to attract it onto the cornea.
- Partially fold lenses to cope with very small palpebral apertures.
- With high plus or aphakic lenses, because of the effect of gravity it may be easier to insert lenses with the head horizontal.
- With difficult, tight-lidded patients it is sometimes much easier to insert the left lens first, since the angle of approach is better.

Once the lens is correctly centred, the patient should notice only slight lid sensation. Any significant discomfort is probably due to a foreign body either carried in with the lens or already present in the tear film and subsequently trapped. The lens should be removed, rinsed and reinserted. Mild discomfort, which patients may describe as stinging, is frequently cured by sliding the lens onto the temporal sclera with a circular motion and allowing it to recentre.

REMOVAL

Removal is effected either by pinching from the temporal or inferior sclera, or by applying lid pressure in a similar way to hard lenses.

Practical advice

● Hard lens scissors methods can be tried with soft lenses, but because of their softness and size they do not always prove effective, particularly if ultra-thin.

● Because of osmotic imbalance, a lens may sometimes appear to stick to the cornea. The eye should be irrigated with 0.9% normal saline and after a short while the lens may be drawn gently onto the sclera and removed.

References

1. Sheridan, M. (1987) Aids virus in tears. *The Optician*, **193**(5083), 15
2. Buckley, R.J. (1991) Acanthamoeba in perspective. Guest Editorial. *Journal of the British Contact Lens Association*, **14**, 5–7.
3. Ficker, L. (1988) Acanthamoeba keratitis – the quest for a better prognosis. *Eye*, **2** (suppl.), s37–s45

Chapter 5

Lens types and materials

5.1 Hard lenses

Hard lens materials are now given the suffix '-focon' and are classified according to the Chemical Groups shown in Table 5.1 [1].

Table 5.1 Chemical Group classification of hard lens (focon) materials (By courtesy of the Association of Contact Lens Manufacturers)

Group 1a
Essentially pure polymethyl methacrylate (99.0%). *Dk* essentially zero.

Group 1b
Copolymers of PMMA with not more than 10% max. of other monomers that may alter hardness, wettability and stability. *Dk* essentially zero.

Group 2a
Essentially pure cellulose acetate butyrate (90%). *Dk* range typically of 2–8.

Group 2b
Copolymers of mixtures of cellulose acetate butyrate and other monomers.

Group 3
Copolymers of one or more alkyl methacrylates with one or more siloxanylmethacrylates, plus other water active monomers and cross-linking agents. Typical *Dk* of more than 6.

Group 4
Hard lens material formed from polysiloxanes.

Group 5
Copolymers of one or more alkyl methacrylates and/or siloxanylmethacrylates, plus other water active monomers, cross-linking agents, and at least 5% by weight of a fluoroalkyl methacrylate or other fluorine containing monomers. Typical *Dk* of more than 20.

Hard lenses are therefore available in a wide range of materials and *Dk* values. Oxygen considerations, however, must take into account the barrier effect which reduces the *Dk* on the eye to approximately 55% of that measured in air [2], together with centre and average lens thickness [3,4].

For physiological reasons lenses should be as thin as possible, but in practical terms making lenses too thin is counter-productive since they are very likely to distort throughout the power range and also become too brittle. In most cases, a realistic minimum centre thickness is 0.14 mm even for high minus powers.

Although Dk is important, there are several other considerations which affect comfort, vision and life span. These include:

- Lens design.
- Fitting method.
- Manufacturing technique.
- Mechanical stability.
- Optical quality.
- Surface wetting properties.

5.1.1 Cellulose acetate butyrate

Cellulose acetate butyrate (CAB) was one of the first modern hard lens materials, introduced in 1977. By modern standards its Dk (between 4 and 8×10^{-11}) is low and it is now less often fitted as the lens of first choice. Its main difficulty when manufactured by traditional lathing methods is dimensional instability. However, when manufactured by moulding, this problem has been largely overcome and lenses such as Conflex and Persecon E give very good clinical results.

ADVANTAGES

- Good wettability.
- Relatively inert.
- Does not attract protein.
- Low breakage rate.
- Very low incidence of papillary conjunctivitis (PC).
- Relatively good for 3 and 9 o'clock staining.

DISADVANTAGES

- Moulding necessary for dimensional stability.
- Limited range of lens designs.
- Scratches easily.

- Attracts lipids from the tears.
- Corneal adhesion in some cases.
- Lens flexure and distortion on toric corneas with tight lids.

Practical advice

CAB is very useful as a problem solver:

- With PC, where contact lens wear can generally be maintained while the condition resolves.
- Where other materials with different wetting properties cause severe 3 and 9 o'clock staining.

5.1.2 Silicone acrylates (siloxanes)

Silicone acrylates are copolymers in varying proportions of acrylate (PMMA) which provides lens rigidity and silicone which controls the degree of oxygen permeability. An excellent range of materials is now available with widely different physical properties and Dk values (see Table 5.2 for examples). They give a superior oxygen and physiological performance compared with CAB, and most have stood the test of time in terms of dimensional stability and optical and mechanical results. They are routinely fitted for daily use and to a limited degree for extended wear.

Table 5.2 Silicone acrylates

Lens	Dk at 35°C
Polycon II	12
Boston II	15
XL40	15
Boston IV	26.7
GP 50	50
Persecon CE	54
Paraperm EW	56

ADVANTAGES

- Wide range of materials available.
- Wide range of designs with practitioner control.

- Medium to high Dks available.
- Good dimensional stability.
- Good vision with limited lens flexure.
- Less easily scratched.

DISADVANTAGES

- Attract protein from the tears.
- Some materials are brittle with a breakage problem.
- High incidence of 3 and 9 o'clock staining.
- Some incidence of PC.

5.1.3 Fluorosilicone acrylates and fluoropolymers

This newer generation of materials is based mainly on fluorine (Table 5.3) [5].

Fluoropolymers incorporate fluorine into the polymer chain to improve oxygen permeability, wettability and deposit resistance. The 3M Fluorofocon A, for example, also includes N-vinyl pyrrolidone (NVP) for its surface-wetting properties and methyl methacrylate for additional strength and stiffness.

Fluorosilicone acrylates are copolymers of silicone, fluorocarbon and methyl methacrylate.

Table 5.3 Fluorine based polymers

Lens	Dk at 35°C
Boston RXD	45
Conflex Air	52
Menicon EX	52
Equalens	71
Fluoroperm	92
Persecon	92
Quantum	92
3M (Advent)	170

ADVANTAGES

- Very high Dks possible.
- Suitable for flexible extended wear.
- Good wettability.
- Fewer deposit problems.

- Low incidence of PC.
- Easy to modify.

DISADVANTAGES

- Brittle if too thin.
- Require careful manufacture.
- Dimensional stability depends on material and manufacture.
- Corneal adhesion in some cases.

General advice

- CAB lenses are suitable where a low *Dk* is sufficient, and where PC and 3 and 9 o'clock staining are a problem with other materials.
- Low *Dk* silicone acrylates are suitable for most straight-forward patients and give good dimensional stability.
- High *Dk* silicone acrylate lenses are suitable for normal daily wear and for most problem solving, with the exception of PC. They are feasible but not ideal for extended wear.
- Fluorosilicone acrylates are better at most problem solving, including PC. They are also equally suitable for either straightforward daily use or flexible extended wear.

5.2 Polymethyl methacrylate (PMMA)

Polymethyl methacrylate (PMMA) has been in use since the 1940s, first as a replacement for the earlier glass scleral lenses, and subsequently as the material of choice with the development of corneal lenses. There are now large numbers of patients who have successfully worn PMMA for 25 years and longer. It is now falling into disuse with the advent of modern hard lenses, by comparison with which its permeability is negligible. However, its original merits of inertness and stability mean that it retains a place for a tiny minority of new patients. There are also many long-standing patients who exhibit neither signs nor symptoms and are best left without refitting, although their corneas should be carefully monitored.

5.2.1 Modified PMMA

Although PMMA has relatively good surface-wetting properties by comparison with many hard lens materials, various versions with modified surface properties (e.g. BP-flex) have been introduced. The improved wettability can give moderately better comfort and the increased tear flow beneath the lens has been beneficial in reducing some of the oedema problems inevitable with an almost impermeable material.

5.3 Soft lenses

Soft lenses are generally discussed according to the interrelated properties of water content, Dk and material type. Materials are now given the suffix '-filcon' and are classified according to the Chemical Groups shown in Table 5.4 [1].

Table 5.4 Chemical Group classification of soft lens (filcon) materials (By courtesy of the Association of Contact Lens Manufacturers)

Group 1a
Essentially pure 2-hydroxyethyl methacrylate (HEMA), containing not more than 0.2% weight of any ionizable chemical (e.g. methacrylic acid).

Group 1b
Essentially pure 2-hydroxyethyl methacrylate, containing more than 0.2% weight of any ionizable chemical.

Group 2a
A copolymer of 2-hydroxyethyl methacrylate and/or other hydroxyalkyl methacrylates, dihydroxyalkylmethacrylates and alkyl methacrylates, but not more than 0.2% weight of any ionizable chemicals.

Group 2b
As described in Group 2a, but containing more than 0.2% weight of any ionizable chemicals.

Group 3a
A copolymer of 2-hydroxyethyl methacrylate with an N-vinyl lactam and/or an alkyl acrylamide, but containing not more than 0.2% weight of any ionizable chemicals.

Group 3b
As described in Group 3a, but containing more than 0.2% weight of any ionizable chemicals.

Group 4a
A copolymer of alkyl methacrylate and N-vinyl lactam and/or an alkyl acrylamide, but containing not more than 0.2% weight of any ionizable chemicals.

Group 4b
As described in Group 4a, but containing more than 0.2% weight of any ionizable chemicals.

Group 5
Soft lens materials formed from polysiloxanes.

WATER CONTENT AND WATER UPTAKE

The definitions for water content and uptake are given in Section 1.3.2. Care must be exercised when interpreting brand names which include a numerical suffix, because these do not always accurately reflect the true water content.

IONIC AND NON-IONIC POLYMERS

Polymers can also be categorized into four groups by linking water content to ionic properties. It is a materials rather than a clinical classification, but generally ionic polymers contain methacrylic acid and attract greater levels of deposit from the tears.

(1) Low water content, non-ionic polymers, e.g. Crofilcon (CSI), 38.5%.

(2) High water content, non-ionic polymers, e.g. Lidofilcon-A (B & L, 70%).

(3) Low water content, ionic polymers, e.g. Bufilcon-A (Hydrocurve II, 45%).

(4) High water content, ionic polymers, e.g. Etafilcon-A (Acuvue, 58%).

5.3.1 Clinical implications of soft lens water content

Lenses have been produced with water contents from 3% to 85%. However, a great many of the lenses currently being used are still hydroxymethyl methacrylate (HEMA)-based, in the region of 38–45%.

ADVANTAGES OF LOW WATER CONTENT LENSES

● Greater tensile strength.

● Less breakage.

● Longer life span.

● Smaller swell factor.

● Better reproducibility.

● Easier to manufacture.

● Can be made thinner.

● Less dehydration on the eye.

● Less discolouration with age.

● Fewer solutions problems.

DISADVANTAGES OF LOW WATER CONTENT LENSES

The disadvantages of low water content lenses relate mainly to the relatively low *Dk* values:

● A greater tendency to cause oedema.
● A long-term tendency with thicker lenses to cause vascularization.

ADVANTAGES OF HIGH WATER CONTENT LENSES

Most high water content materials have *Dk*s between three and five times that of HEMA. Apart from their obvious application in oedema cases, they have several other advantages:

● Better comfort because of material softness.
● Faster adaptation.
● Longer wearing time.
● Extended wear.
● Easier to handle because of greater thickness.
● Better vision because of greater thickness.
● Better for intermittent wear.

DISADVANTAGES OF HIGH WATER CONTENT LENSES

Despite these good features, there are nevertheless disadvantages with high water content lenses which preclude their use in some cases:

● Shorter life span.
● Greater fragility.
● More deposits, especially white spots.
● More discolouration.
● Reproducibility less reliable.
● More difficult to manufacture.
● Greater variation with environment.
● Fitting requires longer settling time.
● Greater variability with vision.
● More solutions problems.

● Corneal desiccation.

● Lens dehydration.

5.3.2 Clinical implications of soft lens thickness

The typical centre thickness for a 'standard' corneal diameter HEMA lens of power −3.00 D is in the region of 0.10–0.14 mm. Lenses below 0.10 mm may be regarded as 'thin'; those below 0.07 mm as 'ultra-thin' and thinner than 0.05 mm as 'hyper-thin'. They represent a very satisfactory way of increasing transmissibility (Dk/t) and improving physiological performance, as well as giving an inherent safety factor for patients who accidentally fall asleep while wearing their lenses. Low plus and aphakic lenses cannot truly be considered ultra-thin because of their necessarily greater centre thickness. Nevertheless, 'thin' plus lenses give a more satisfactory result.

Oxygen performance for a lens cannot be judged solely in relation to its specified centre thickness, but must be considered for the entire lens. If an 'average' or 'mean' thickness is used, this itself requires definition to avoid error and give valid comparison [6].

ADVANTAGES OF THIN LENSES

● Lower incidence of oedema.

● Reduced lid sensation because of thinner edges.

● Reduced limbal irritation because of thinner edges and larger total diameter.

● Different fitting characteristic may provide better centration than standard lenses.

● Easier to fit because fewer fitting steps are necessary.

● Safer if patients accidentally fall asleep.

DISADVANTAGES OF THIN LENSES

● Handling is more difficult, especially in low minus powers below about −2.00 D.

● Higher breakage rate than standard thickness lenses.

● Life span is shorter, especially with heat disinfection.

● Visual acuity may be less good with toric corneas.

● Greater tendency to dehydrate on the eye and disturb precorneal tear film.

5.3.3 Dehydration of soft lenses

One of the major reasons for the clinical success or failure of a particular lens on the eye relates to its dehydration characteristics.

EFFECTS OF LENS DEHYDRATION

- Change in parameters and fitting.
- Reduced comfort.
- Reduced *Dk*.
- Disruption of tear film.
- Corneal desiccation and staining.
- Increased deposits.
- Reduced vision.

FACTORS INFLUENCING LENS DEHYDRATION

Ocular factors

- Volume of tears.
- Quality and stability of tear film.
- Osmolarity of tears.
- Blinking habits.
- Size of palpebral aperture.

Other factors

- Lens material.
- Lens thickness.
- Temperature.
- Relative humidity.
- Draughts and wind.
- Systemic drugs.
- Alcohol.

The water content contained within the polymer matrix consists of 'bound' water directly attached to hydrophilic sites by van der Waals' forces and 'free' water which is readily lost by evaporation. The higher the bound water, the less any particular material will dehydrate on the eye [7].

Generally, most water loss occurs within the first few minutes and high water content materials give greater dehydration. Tear film stability is better with thicker lenses and low water contents: it is worse with ultra-thin and high water content lenses.

5.4 Silicone lenses

5.4.1 Silicone rubber lenses

Silicone lenses differ from hard lenses in several ways. They can be flexed, stretched and turned inside out. They have excellent elastic properties, partly conform to the shape of the cornea in wear, and have extremely high Dks, in the region of 200×10^{-11}. They are also unlike hydrophilic lenses because their natural state is dry and they are extremely tough. Since they do not absorb water to any significant extent, fluorescein can be used in their fitting and they do not need disinfecting in the same way as soft lenses.

Because of the amorphous nature of the silicone rubber raw materials, lenses are produced by a moulding and vulcanization technique, which also assists in maintaining good reproducibility. The main difficulty with silicone is that its natural surface is extremely hydrophobic, and it has been necessary to devise methods of rendering the surface permanently hydrophilic without interfering with any of its optical or physical properties. The final stage of manufacture is therefore surface treatment by ion bombardment.

Because of the following advantages and disadvantages, silicone has remained very much a minority lens with limited therapeutic applications (*see* Section 31.3).

ADVANTAGES OF SILICONE LENSES

- Very high Dk.
- Better and more stable vision than many soft lenses.
- Little variation in comfort or fitting with environmental factors.
- Low risk of loss or damage.

DISADVANTAGES OF SILICONE LENSES

- Difficult to fit, requiring as much precision as hard lenses.

- A negative pressure effect, giving sticking, particularly if not correctly fitted.
- Breakdown in surface coating and difficulties with wetting.
- Build-up of deposits.
- Foreign bodies, especially with loose fittings.

5.4.2 Silicone resin lenses

Resin lenses differ from silicone elastomers because they are not flexible, having many of the physical properties of hard lenses. *Dk* values, however, are significantly lower than elastomers and they have so far found only limited application.

5.5 Other lenses

Soft-coated hard lenses

Aquasil and Novalens (Ocutec) are hard lenses with a 0.005 μm 'soft' coating of OH groups which gives the characteristics of a hydrophilic lens. The lens does not absorb water, but has a good surface wettability and improved comfort. The *Dk* is 55×10^{-11} and lenses are fitted according to hard lens criteria.

Styrene lenses

The Wesley–Jessen Airlens is produced from *t*-butyl styrene which contains no silicone. The material has a *Dk* of 24 at 35°C and a high refractive index of $n = 1.525$. Solutions containing chlorhexidine should be avoided, since they may interfere with the wetting angle of 54°.

Collagen lenses

Collagen lenses are produced from biological polymers and one of the reasons for their development is biocompatibility. Their main applications have been therapeutic.

References

1. Parker, J. (1990) The classification of contact lens materials. In *Contact Lens Year Book 1990*, Medical and Scientific Publishing, Hythe, Kent, p.54
2. Holden, B.A., La Hood, D. and Sweeney, D.F. (1985) Does *Dk/L* measurement accurately predict overnight edema response? *American Journal of Physiological Optics*, **62**, 95P

3. Fatt, I. (1986) Some comments on methods used for measuring oxygen permeability (*Dk*) of contact lens materials. *Contact Lens Association of Ophthalmologists Journal*, **11**, 221–226

4. Brennan, N., Efron, N.A. and Holden, B.A. (1986) Oxygen transmissibility of hard gas permeable and hydrophilic contact lenses. *American Journal of Physiological Optics*, **63**, 4P

5. Fatt, I. (1985) A new look at fluoropolymers. *Optician*, **190**(5015), 25–26

6. Sammons, W.A. (1980) Contact lens thickness and all that. *Optician*, **180**(4467), 11–18

7. Hart, D.E. (1987) Surface interactions on hydrogel contact lenses: scanning electron microscopy (SEM). *Journal of the American Optometric Association*, **58**, 962–974

8. Hill, R.M. (1966) Effects of a silicone rubber contact lens on corneal respiration. *Journal of the American Optometric Association*, **37**, 1119–1121

9. Roth, H.W., Iwaski, W., Takayama, M. and Wada, C. (1980) Complications caused by silicone elastomer lenses in West Germany and Japan. *Contacto*, **24**, 28–36

Chapter 6

Principles of hard and PMMA lens design

6.1 Basic principles of corneal lens design

- Lenses may be spherical, aspheric or a combination of both.
- Most corneal lenses have a central zone which is fitted just apically clear or aligns with the central cornea, combined with a much flatter peripheral zone which is designed to lift away from the cornea.
- Central alignment gives optimum acuity (*see* Section 8.6).
- Peripheral clearance is necessary for adequate tears exchange.
- The transition between the central portion and the periphery is sharp for a spherical bicurve design, becoming smoother as additional curves are added.
- Aspheric lenses have a much smoother transition and for some designs can be compared with very well-blended spherical multicurves (*see* Section 10).

6.2 Forces controlling design

Corneal lenses of all materials are affected by a variety of forces when placed on the eye. These factors are both ocular (*see* Chapter 3) and physical in nature.

6.2.1 Centre of gravity

- The centre of gravity of a lens lies somewhere behind the back surface (Figure 6.1).
- It is affected by radius, diameter, thickness and power.
- Steep lenses have the centre of gravity further back than flat lenses and therefore give better centration (Figure 6.2a).

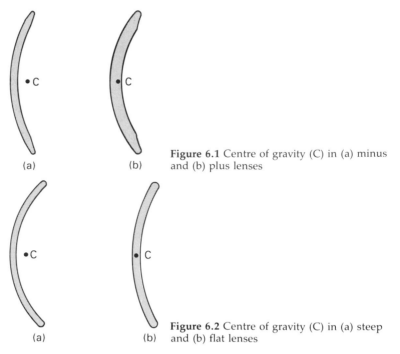

Figure 6.1 Centre of gravity (C) in (a) minus and (b) plus lenses

Figure 6.2 Centre of gravity (C) in (a) steep and (b) flat lenses

- Flat lenses have the centre of gravity further forward and give worse centration (Figure 6.2b).
- Large diameter lenses have the centre of gravity further back than small lenses and give better centration.
- Small lenses have the centre of gravity further forward and give worse centration.

6.2.2 Frictional forces

The viscosity of the tear film maintains the lens in a stationary position by means of frictional forces. Thinning of the tear film or an increase in its aqueous content (e.g. during adaptation) reduces the centration ability of these forces.

6.2.3 Capillary attraction

- The closer the lens matches the shape of the cornea, the greater the capillary attraction and stability.
- Since a hard lens cannot ever exactly match the shape of the cornea, a balance has to be found between sufficient capillary

attraction for lens stability and sufficient movement for tears exchange.

- An excessively flat fitting gives less capillary attraction and greater movement.
- A steep fitting can create a negative pressure or suction effect.
- The tears meniscus at the edge of the lens also provides forces for centration. The greater the meniscus, the better the adhesion.

6.2.4 Specific gravity

- The clinical significance is demonstrated when two lenses of the same design (and volume) but different specific gravity behave differently on the eye. The lens with the lower specific gravity has less weight.
- A lens that drops because gravitational forces are greater than fluid forces may achieve better centration by using a material of lower specific gravity and *vice versa*.
- With prism ballast, a high specific gravity material is advantageous as it gives a greater difference in weight between the apex and base of the lens.

6.2.5 Thickness and lenticulation

Thickness depends on back vertex power (BVP), design and material. Centre thickness (t_c) and edge thickness (t_e) are both important (Tables 6.1 and 6.2).

Table 6.1 Typical thickness values

BVP (D)	t_c (mm)	t_e (mm)
−10.00	0.13	0.25
−6.00	0.13	0.22
−3.00	0.15	0.20
−1.00	0.18	0.18
+1.00	0.22	0.12
+3.00	0.26	0.13
+6.00	0.34	0.15
+10.00	0.45	0.16

Table 6.2 Typical thickness variations for different materials (BVP −3.00 D)

Material	t_c (mm)	t_e (mm)
PMMA	0.10	0.12
CAB	0.16	0.12
Silicone acrylate	0.15	0.13
Fluoropolymer*	0.14	0.15

*Some fluoropolymers can be made as thin as 0.05 mm.

- BVPs greater than −6.00 D or +4.00 D should be lenticulated to reduce excess thickness and mass.

- Lenticulation reduces thickness in the centre for plus and towards the edge for minus lenses by making the front optic zone diameter (FOZD) smaller (Figure 6.3).

- The FOZD should be approximately 0.50 mm larger than the back optic zone diameter (BOZD).

- The carrier portion of a lenticulated lens can be plano, negative or positive in shape (Figure 6.4). The choice

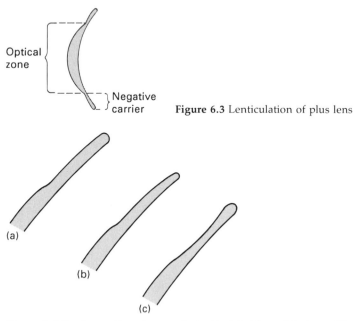

Optical zone

Negative carrier

Figure 6.3 Lenticulation of plus lens

(a)

(b)

(c)

Figure 6.4 Carrier portion shapes of a lenticulated lens: (a) plano; (b) positive; (c) negative

depends upon the intended effect (e.g. lid attachment techniques) (*see* Section 6.5).

Practical advice

- Do not order centre thickness less than 0.14 mm with most modern materials because of lens flexure, particularly with toric corneas and tight lids.
- Edge thickness should be a minimum of 0.12 mm. A 'knife edge' causes discomfort and is fragile, especially with plus lenses.
- Minus lenses usually give a natural lid attachment.
- A negative carrier helps give lid attachment with a low-riding or plus lens.
- A positive carrier helps reduce a high-riding tendency.

6.2.6 Refractive index of materials

The following are typical examples of refractive index:

PMMA: 1.49
CAB: 1.47
Silicone acrylate: 1.471–1.48
Fluoropolymer: 1.439–1.471
Silicone: 1.43

- The higher the refractive index, the thinner the lens can be made.
- Most hard lenses have a lower refractive index than PMMA and are therefore thicker.
- High refractive index plastics are used for bifocal segments. They can incorporate fluorescent dye to assist fitting.
- The refractive index is important in toric lens fitting (*see* Chapter 21).

6.2.7 Edge shape

- Extremely important for comfort.
- Must be smooth and well finished.
- Should blend into the final peripheral curve.
- Can help lens removal.

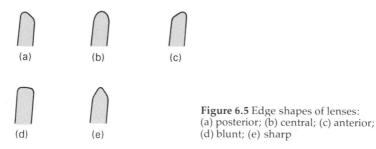

Figure 6.5 Edge shapes of lenses:
(a) posterior; (b) central; (c) anterior;
(d) blunt; (e) sharp

- Varying degrees of taper and roundness are used, depending on fitting philosophy (*see* Section 6.5) and lid sensitivity. Edges are described as (a) posterior, (b) central, (c) anterior, (d) blunt, and (e) sharp (Figure 6.5).
- Edge thickness depends on BVP (*see* Section 6.2.5).

6.3 Concept of edge lift

The concept of edge lift embodies not only the actual edge of the lens, but also the series of peripheral curves which lead into the edge shape.

Current lens designs are usually defined in respect of axial edge lift (AEL). Historically, however, the concept of edge lift has used a variety of terms;

- 'Z value' or axial edge lift.
- Constant axial edge lift (*see* Chapter 7).
- 'Z factor' or radial edge lift.
- Flattening factor.
- Tear layer thickness (*see* Section 6.4).

The 'Z value' or axial edge fit (AEL) is the distance between the posterior surface of the lens and the continuation of the BOZR measured parallel to the primary axis of the lens (Figure 6.6) [1]. It is *not* the distance between the lens and cornea. The usual value of edge lift varies between 0.09 mm and 0.15 mm and rather more for PMMA.

If the same absolute values are given to the peripheral curves of both steep and flat lenses, the steep lens has, relatively, a greater edge lift [2]. Example:

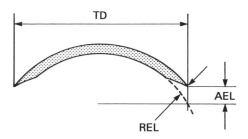

Figure 6.6 Axial edge lift (AEL) and radial edge lift (REL) in a rigid lens design (TD, total diameter)

r $r + 0.5$ $r + 2.2$ $r + 4.7$
8.40:7.00/8.90:8.00/10.60:8.50/13.10:9.00 AEL = 0.117 mm

7.20:7.00/7.70:8.00/9.40:8.50/ 11.90:9.00 AEL = 0.172 mm

CAEL lenses [2] are multicurves which for a given diameter are designed to give the same AEL throughout the range of radii. The clinical appearance and performance are therefore consistent.

The 'Z factor' [3] or radial edge lift (REL) is the distance between the continuation of the BOZR and the final peripheral curve measure normal to the lens edge (Figure 6.6).

The ratio of axial to radial edge lift is approximately 5:4. Example:

7.40:7.00/8.10:7.80/9.30:8.60/10.50:9.00
Taken from 0.15 mm CAEL trial set with a total diameter (TD) of 9.00 mm [2].
AEL at 7.80 = 0.025
AEL at 8.60 = 0.095
AEL at 9.00 = 0.15 The designated value for the final peri
                    pheral curve
REL at 9.00 = 0.120 Ratio REL/AEL = 0.80

The flattening factor (ff) defines the extent to which the peripheral curve flattens in relation to the central radius in an offset lens (*see* Section 7.2).

6.3.1 Function of edge lift and edge clearance

The lens periphery must be fitted significantly flatter than the cornea to:

● Provide tears exchange beneath the lens for the maintenance of corneal metabolism.

- Give a tears meniscus so that capillary attraction and lens centration forces can function (*see* Section 6.2).
- Assist lens removal by the lids.
- Avoid pressure and corneal insult at the lens edge.
- Avoid lens adhesion.

N.B. AEL relates to the lens design off the eye. Edge clearance relates to the lens on the eye.

6.3.2 Designs of edge lift

Edge lift and peripheral clearance depend on corneal topography and lens design. Too little edge clearance lift gives.

- Inadequate tears exchange.
- Poor lens movement.
- Pressure at the lens edge and arcuate staining.
- Difficulty with lens removal.
- Lens adhesion.

Too much edge clearance gives:

- Excessive lens movement.
- Bubbles under the lens periphery which can cause frothing or dimpling.
- Poor centration.
- Lens displacement off the cornea.
- 3 and 9 o'clock staining because of tear film disruption.

6.4 Tear layer thickness (TLT)

- Tear layer thickness (TLT) is the clearance between the back surface of the lens and the cornea, usually in respect of the central area. (Typical example Figure 6.7.)
- The fitting technique and lens design govern the values for apical (and edge) clearance.
- TLT is expressed in *micrometres* (μm) (1 μm = 0.001 mm), whereas edge lift is given in millimetres and relates only to the physical dimensions of the lens.

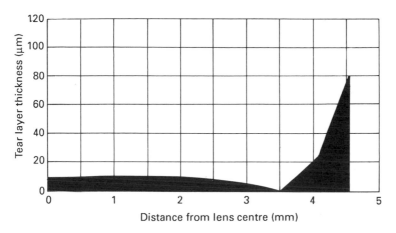

Figure 6.7 Tear layer profile

Typical values [4]

Tear layer thickness = 5–10 μm
Edge clearance (EC)   = 75–80 μm

6.5 Lid attachment lenses

Lid attachment (hitch-up) utilizes the edge contour and shape of the anterior peripheral surface of the lens to increase lid–lens adhesion [5,6].

- Lid attachment occurs when peripheral lens contour remains in constant contact with the upper lid margin after blinking or eye closure.
- The lens therefore moves with the upper lid and returns to a superior position on the cornea after blinking.
- Minus lenses give a natural lid attachment on most eyes because of their edge shape, but larger diameter lenses are often necessary (Figure 6.8).
- When the upper lid is in its normal position, its upward retention effect on the lens is greater than the downwards pull of gravity or the centration forces of the tears meniscus.
- Plus lenses give the reverse effect and tend to escape from lid retention because of their edge shape.
- The correct anterior lenticular construction is essential.

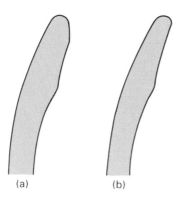

(a)   (b)

Figure 6.8 Korb edge contour (a), compared with a standard edge design (b)

ADVANTAGES

● More comfortable.

● Helps maintain normal blinking.

● Counteracts low riding lenses.

● Helps tears exchange on blinking.

● Lenses can be made thinner with high powers.

● Less 3 and 9 o'clock staining.

DISADVANTAGES

● Flare from lower edge of pupil.

● Peripheral curves may need to be individually designed.

● Front surface may require complex construction.

6.6 Interpalpebral lenses

The technique aims to give good centration using very thin lenses with a total diameter smaller than the vertical palpebral aperture. It has mainly been applied to PMMA to improve the physiological performance and where thinner lenses can be more easily manufactured.

Fitting

TD: At least 2.00 mm larger than maximum pupil diameter, i.e. usually 7.50–8.50 mm.

BOZR: Up to 0.15 mm steeper than flattest 'K' to give the appearance of an alignment fit.

BOZD: 5.00–7.00 mm.

Example 1: 7.80:6.50/8.60:7.50/10.40:8.50 t_c = 0.10

Example 2: 7.80:7.00/10.50:8.00 t_c = 0.08

ADVANTAGES

- Better for narrow lid apertures.
- Less sensation with sensitive lids.
- Better for corneas with irregular periphery.
- Often successful with moderate or even highly toric corneas where a small lens may permit a spherical design.
- Less disturbance of corneal metabolism.
- Lens positions away from the limbus and may help with 3 and 9 o'clock staining or limbal disturbance.

DISADVANTAGES

- More difficult to manufacture because they must be made thinner.
- Difficult to handle.
- Difficult to remove.
- Fragile edges.
- Flare.
- Disincentive to blinking and may give increased 3 and 9 o'clock staining.

References

1. Bennett, A.G. (1968) Aspherical contact lens surfaces. *Ophthalmic Optician*, **8**, 1037–1040, 1297–1300, 1311; **9**, 222–230
2. Stone, J. (1975) Corneal lenses with constant axial edge lift. *Ophthalmic Optician*, **15**, 818–824
3. Hodd, F.A.B. (1966) A design study of the back surface of corneal contact lenses. *Ophthalmic Optician*, **6**, 1175–1178, 1187–1190, 1203, 1229–1232, 1235–1238; **7**, 14–16, 19–21, 39
4. Atkinson, T.C.O. (1987) The development of the back surface design of rigid lenses. *Contax*, Nov., 5–18
5. Korb, D.R. and Korb, J.E. (1970) A new concept in contact lens design. *Journal of the American Optometric Association*, **41**, 1023
6. Mackie, I. (1973) Design compensation in corneal lens fitting. In *Symposium on Contact Lenses: Transactions of the New Orleans Academy of Ophthalmology*, Mosby, St. Louis

Chapter 7
Development of hard lens design

7.1 Introduction

The first PMMA corneal lens was designed in 1947 [1]. It consisted of a single curve approximately 0.30 mm flatter than 'K' and a total diameter of about 11.00 mm. Limited practical success was achieved for physiological reasons. It was not until practitioners such as Bier in the early 1950s realized that the cornea was more complicated than a simple sphere, that a bicurve construction was introduced. Further improvements were made by adding a flatter, third curve to assist tear circulation. The complex elliptical shape of the cornea was more fully understood by the late 1960s and multicurve lenses evolved together with the first aspheric constructions [2]. Most designs were fitted as:

- Either central alignment or minimal clearance with peripheral clearance.
- Central clearance with peripheral alignment.

The following BSI/ISO terminology, abbreviations and symbols are used:

BOZR (r_0) = back optic zone radius
BOZD ($\varnothing_0$) = back optic zone diameter
r_1 = first back peripheral radius
$\varnothing_1$ = first back peripheral zone diameter
r_2 = second back peripheral radius
TD ($\varnothing_T$) = total diameter

In addition, 'K' is used to refer to flattest keratometry reading

7.2 Early lens design

Bier contour technique

Developed in the UK by Bier in 1957 [3]. A spherical bicurve design, fitted with apical alignment and peripheral clearance.

Now rarely used except for refitting existing problem-free wearers.

BOZR = 'K' ± 0.10 mm
r_1 = BOZR + 0.40–0.80 mm
BOZD = 6.50–7.50 mm
TD = 8.50–10.00 mm

Example: 7.80:6.80/8.60:9.65 −3.00 (Figure 7.1)

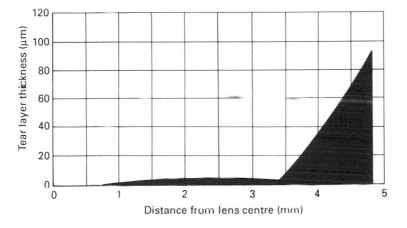

Figure 7.1 Tear layer profile/Bier contour technique

Modified contour technique

A tricurve, modified version of the Bier contour technique. The fitting is central alignment with the first peripheral curve, giving some degree of corneal alignment; the final curve is small and flat. Occasionally used for refitting and where large edge lift is required with PMMA.

BOZR = 'K' ± 0.50 mm
r_1 = BOZR + 0.30–0.50 mm
r_2 = 9.50–12.50 mm, 0.20–0.40 mm wide
BOZD = 6.00–7.50 mm
TD = 8.50–9.50 mm

Example: 7.80:6.50/8.30:9.10/12.25:9.50 −3.00 (Figure 7.2)

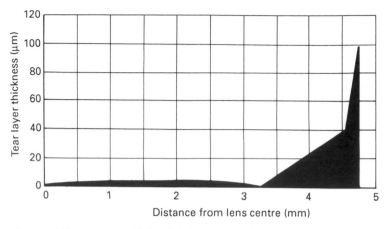

Figure 7.2 Tear layer profile/modified contour technique

Bayshore technique

Developed in the USA by Bayshore in 1962 [4]. A small tricurve corneal lens, fitted to give central clearance and peripheral alignment. Occasionally used to give a tight interpalpebral fitting.

BOZR   = 'K' − 0.30 mm
BOZD   = 5.60–6.60 mm
TD   = 7.00–8.80 mm (0.20 mm less than the vertical palpebral aperture)
r_1 = BOZR + 1.00–1.50 mm (aligned with cornea)
r_2 = 17.00 mm, 0.10–0.30 mm wide
Fenestration = central, 0.20–0.25 mm in diameter

Example: 7.60:6.00/8.80:7.00/17.00:7.60 −3.00
           Single central fenestration, 0.20 mm

Conoid lens

Developed in Australia by Thomas in 1967 [5]. Fitted to give apical clearance, it has a spherical BOZR with a conical periphery commonly tangential to the BOZR.

Comfort is good because of reduced lid sensation, but gross corneal steepening and distortion occurs. Now only used for occasional refitting and where a very tight lens is required for centration.

BOZR   = 'K' − 0.30 mm

BOZD   = 6.50 mm
TD   = 9.00 mm
Fenestration = 0.25 mm in diameter, 0.20 mm in from the lens
             edge, just within the optic zone.

Percon lens

Developed in Holland by Stek in 1969 [6] and in the UK by
Cantor in 1970 [7]. It has a spherical BOZR and a conical
peripheral zone with a constant axial lift of 0.10 mm. The cone
angle is almost exactly tangential to give virtually no transition
(*see* Offset lens, below). The fitting gives central alignment with
peripheral clearance and is occasionally used to give large edge
lift with PMMA.

BOZR   = 'K' + 0.05 mm
BOZD   = 6.60–7.20 mm (related to cone angle)
TD   = 8.60–9.40 mm
Cone angle = depends on both BOZR and TD

Example: 7.80:6.80/ 9.00   Cone angle 130°

Offset lens

Developed in the UK by Ruben in 1966 [8]. The centre of
curvature of the back peripheral curve is offset to the opposite
side of the central axis, virtually eliminating any transition. It
has been termed a 'continuous bicurve lens' [2] or 'Contralateral
offset' (Figure 7.3). A 'homolateral offset' is also possible, where

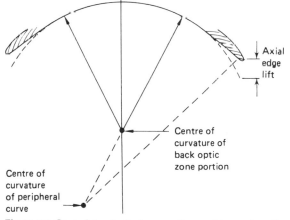

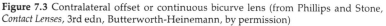
Figure 7.3 Contralateral offset or continuous bicurve lens (from Phillips and Stone,
Contact Lenses, 3rd edn, Butterworth-Heinemann, by permission)

the centre of curvature of the peripheral curve is displaced to the same side of the central axis.

The degree of flattening is referred to as the 'axial edge lift', 'Z value' or 'flattening factor'. It is usually specified by the distance at the lens edge between the extension of the BOZR and the peripheral curve. The distance in millimetres is measured along a line parallel to the axis of symmetry.

Offset lenses give good comfort because of the minimal transition and are useful for early keratoconus and where large edge lift is required with PMMA. The small optic, however, gives flare and special offset lathes are required for manufacture.

Offset No 1   BOZD: 6.00 mm   TD: 9.00 mm
Offset No 2   BOZD: 6.90 mm   TD: 10.00 mm
Offset No 3   BOZD: 5.50 mm   TD: 8.50 mm

All with a flattening factor (AEL) of 0.10 mm in low minus powers.

Example: 7.00:6.00 AEL 0.1 at 9.00   −5.00

7.3 Current designs: bicurve, tricurve, multicurve

Corneal lenses are now designed with one or more peripheral zones which are deliberately intended to lift away from the cornea. Most modern spherical lenses are based on these designs.

Bicurve (C2): Consists of a central radius and one flatter peripheral curve (Figure 7.4). There is a sharp transition between the two curves.

Examples: 7.80:7.00/8.70:9.00 (Figure 7.5)
7.80:7.80/10.50:9.00 (Figure 7.6)

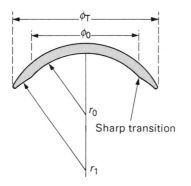

Sharp transition

Figure 7.4 Bicurve corneal lens ($\varnothing_T$, total diameter; $\varnothing_0$, back optic zone diameter; r_0, back optic zone radius; r_1, first back peripheral radius)

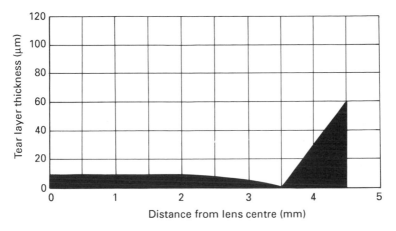

Figure 7.5 Tear layer profile/bicurve (C2)

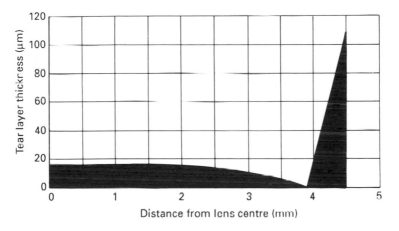

Figure 7.6 Tear layer profile/bicurve (C2)

*Tricurve (C3):*Consists of a central radius and two flatter peripheral curves (Figure 7.7). It is the basic design of most modern hard lenses, where the final curve is much flatter than first peripheral radius.

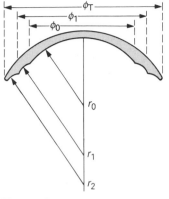

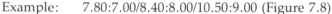

Figure 7.7 Tricurve corneal lens ($\varnothing_T$, total diameter; $\varnothing_1$, first back peripheral zone diameter; $\varnothing_0$, back optic zone diameter; r_0, back optic zone radius; r_1 first back peripheral radius; r_2, second back peripheral radius) (from Phillips and Stone, *Contact Lenses*, 3rd edn, Butterworth-Heinemann, by permission)

Example: 7.80:7.00/8.40:8.00/10.50:9.00 (Figure 7.8)

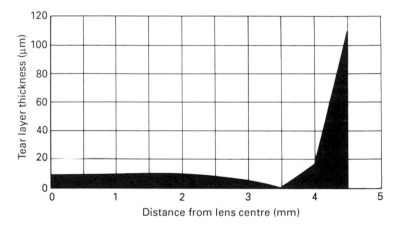

Figure 7.8 Tear layer profile/tricurve (C3)

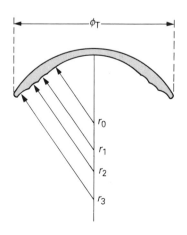

Figure 7.9 Multicurve corneal lens (r_3, third back peripheral radius; other symbols as in Figure 7.4)

Multicurve: Consists of a central radius and three or more peripheral curves (Figure 7.9). It follows the flattening of cornea better than bicurves and tricurves, and when the transitions are well blended, behaves like a continuous curve lens.

Example: 7.80:7.00/8.40:7.90/8.90:8.80/11.25:9.30 (Figure 7.10)

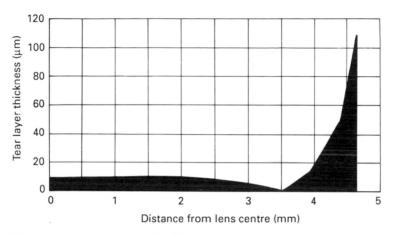

Figure 7.10 Tear layer profile/multicurve

Constant axial edge lift

CAEL lenses [9] (*see* Section 6.3) were developed as a further refinement of multicurve lens design to give a constant linear clearance between the edge of the lens and the cornea, over the whole range of radii for a given diameter. The axial edge lift of the peripheral curves is calculated to remain constant for all BOZRs, unlike conventional lenses where the calculated AEL is greater with steeper lenses than with flatter lenses.

N.B. AEL relates to the lens design off the eye.

Average CAEL for a TD of 8.60 mm ≡ 0.105 mm
Average CAEL for a TD of 9.20 mm ≡ 0.11 mm
Average CAEL for a TD of 9.60 mm ≡ 0.14 mm

7.4 Aspheric lenses

Aspheric lenses have one or both surfaces of a non-spherical construction. Aspherics usually take the form of a parabola, ellipse or hyperbola and are defined by eccentricity.

DEFINITIONS

Eccentricity (e):   Defines mathematically the departure of an aspheric curve from a circle. Used to describe both a lens form and the curvature of the cornea.

'P value':   Defines the rate of flattening with eccentricity: $P = 1 - e^2$.

The closest mathematical approximation to the topography of the human cornea is an ellipse. Mean eccentricity = 0.45; $P = 0.8$.

Circle: Completely symmetrical. Eccentricity = 0; $P = 1$.

Ellipse: Symmetrical about two axes, but has two diameters – one long and one short. Eccentricity = $0 < E < 1$; $P = <1$.

Parabola: Symmetrical about one axis. Eccentricity = 1; $P = 0$.

Hyperbola: Eccentricity >1; $P = <0$.

7.4.1 Aspheric designs

Nissel aspheric

The Nissel design (1967) [10], now rarely used, was based on the USA Volk lens. It has a central aspheric portion with a 7.80 mm diameter; two spherical zones at diameters of 8.40 mm and 8.80 mm; and an 0.50 mm wide bevel of 10.00–12.00 mm to prevent corneal indentation and assist tear flow. It is fitted to give central corneal alignment with the appearance of a multicurve.

BOZR (aspheric) = 'K' − 0.10 mm
BOZD   = 7.80 mm
$\varnothing_1$ = 8.40 mm
TD   = 8.80 mm
Typical 'Z values' = 0.075 mm at 8.00 mm
                     0.115 mm at 9.50 mm

Conflex (Wohlk, 1982)

Moulded from Anduran material (CAB + ethyl vinyl acetate), this lens [11] consists of a spherical optic with three aspheric peripheral zones. The edge shape is termed 'ski-tip'. The lens is fitted 2.00 mm less than the horizontal visible iris diameter (HVID) to give central alignment, or just flatter than 'K' with slight superior decentration.

TD   = 9.40 mm, 9.90 mm, 10.20 mm
BOZR   = 'K' + 0.00–0.10 mm
Aspheric periphery = 0.80 mm, 1.60 mm, 3.50 mm flatter than
                       BOZR

Conflex air (Wohlk, 1989)

A fully aspheric design in a fluoropolymer material, fitted with central alignment.

TD   = 9.30 mm, 9.80 mm, 10.30 mm
BOZR   = 7.20–8.60 mm
Aspheric periphery = (e = 0.4)

Persecon E (CIBA, 1981)

The aspheric version of an earlier spherical design, both in CAB. The back surface gradually flattens to the periphery with e = 0.40 and P = 0.84. There is a spherical edge curve to assist tears exchange. It is fitted to give minimum edge clearance either with central alignment or slightly flat to ensure adequate movement and tears exchange.

BOZR   = 'K' + 0.10 mm
Spherical edge width   = 0.20–0.30 mm
Spherical peripheral radius = 10.00–12.00 mm
TD   = 8.80 mm, 9.30 mm, 9.80 mm,
                                  10.30 mm
Edge clearance   = 20–60 μm

TD (mm)	AEL (mm)
8.80	0.016–0.030
9.30	0.020–0.041
9.80	0.025–0.053
10.30	0.033–0.069

References

1. Dickenson, F. and Hall, K.G.C. (1946) *An Introduction to the Prescribing and Fitting of Contact Lenses*, Hammond and Hammond, London
2. Bennett, A.G. (1968) Aspherical contact lens surfaces. *Ophthalmic Optician*, **8**, 1037–1040, 1297–1300, 1311; **9**, 222–230
3. Bier, N. (1957) The contour lens. *Journal of the American Optometric Association*, **28**, 394–396
4. Bayshore, C.A. (1962) Report on 276 patients fitted with microcorneal lenses apical clearance and central ventilation. *American Journal of Optometry*, **39**, 552–553

5. Thomas, P.F. (1967) *Conoid Contact Lenses*, Corneal Lens Corporation, Australia
6. Stek, A.W. (1969) The Percon contact lens – design and fitting technique. *Contact Lens*, **2**, 12–14
7. Cantor, D. (1970) The Percon lens – design and fitting techniques. In *Fitting Manual*, Darling and Cantor Ltd, Brackley, Northants
8. Ruben, M. (1966) Use of conoidal curves in corneal contact lenses. *British Journal of Ophthalmology*, **50**, 642–645
9. Stone, J. (1975) Corneal lenses with constant axial edge lift. *Ophthalmic Optician*, **15**, 818–824
10. Nissel, G. (1967) Aspheric contact lenses. *Ophthalmic Optician*, **7**, 1007–1010
11. Gasson, A.P. (1982) Conflex, a new gas permeable hard lens. *Optician*, **184**, 25–29

Chapter 8

Hard lens selection and fitting

8.1 Introduction

Compared with PMMA, modern hard lenses can employ different fitting criteria because of:

- The physical properties of the materials (e.g. flexibility).
- Oxygen transmission and the improved physiological response of the cornea.
- The problems it is hoped they will solve (e.g. flare).

8.2 Back optic zone radius (BOZR)

- Trial sets usually have steps of 0.10 mm, although prescription lenses can normally be ordered in 0.05 mm steps.
- The preferred fitting for most corneal lenses is alignment or very slightly flatter.
- Trial lens selection is based on keratometry.
- The initial lens usually has a BOZR nearest to flattest 'K'.
- Toric corneas (1.00–3.00 D of astigmatism) should also be fitted on or near flattest 'K' to minimize flexure and achieve good acuity with a spherical lens [1].
- The radius must be considered in relation to BOZD. Where a very large optic is required (e.g. 8.40 mm), the radius is usually flatter (e.g. 'K' + 0.10 mm) to achieve an alignment fitting.
- Additional factors such as lid tension, BVP and centre of gravity must also be considered (*see* Section 6.2).

● Right and left eyes generally require radii within 0.05 mm of each other, except in cases of anisometropia.

Example 1   (Alignment): 'K' 8.00 × 7.95
              Initial radius selected: 8.00 mm
Example 2:   (Alignment): 'K' 7.97 × 7.83
              Initial radius selected: 8.00 mm
Example 3:   (Toric cornea): 'K' 8.00 × 7.50
              Initial radius selected: 7.95 mm

8.3 Total diameter (TD)

● Compared with PMMA, it is possible to err on the large side, since the material and lens design provide the necessary oxygen and tear flow.

● TD is chosen on the basis of corneal size to be approximately 2.0 mm smaller than HVID.

● TD depends on pupil size, especially in low illumination.

● TD depends on the size of vertical palpebral aperture.

● The choice can be regarded as *small* (<9.20 mm), *medium* (9.20–9.70 mm) or *large* (>9.80 mm).

● Changing to a larger diameter generally stabilizes the fitting, although it does not always have a significant effect on the fluorescein pattern.

● Highly toric corneas need either small lenses to avoid excessive edge stand-off in the steep meridian or large lenses for lid attachment.

● The TD should be evaluated in relation to BVP. High powers require larger diameters for lens stability.

● The final choice of diameter also depends on the method of fitting (e.g. whether lid attachment or interpalpebral).

● Right and left eyes almost always require the same TD.

8.4 Back optic zone diameter (BOZD)

● Often predetermined by the laboratory.

● Depends on pupil size, especially in low illumination.

- The pupil position must be assessed for aphakics.
- BOZD is chosen to be at least 1.50 mm larger than pupil size.
- The choice may be regarded as *small* (<7.30 mm), *medium* (7.30–7.90 mm) or *large* (>7.90 mm).
- A larger BOZD for a particular radius gives a greater sag and therefore a steeper fitting.
- A smaller BOZD is often chosen with a toric cornea to reduce the area of mismatch.
- A larger BOZD is often chosen to permit a flatter BOZR which gives less flexure on a toric cornea.
- An excessively large BOZD gives a periphery which is very narrow. The peripheral curves must therefore be much flatter than normal for adequate edge clearance. This results in a sharp transition.
- The BOZD should be considered in relation to BVP and lenticulation. High minus lenses frequently require very large BOZDs to avoid flare.

Typical fittings:

Example 1: 7.80:7.50/8.60:8.30/10.50:9.30 (Figure 8.1)

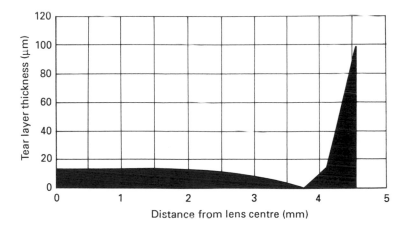

Figure 8.1 Tear layer profile/BOZD

Example 2: 7.80:8.20/8.70:8.90/10.50:9.80 (Figure 8.2)

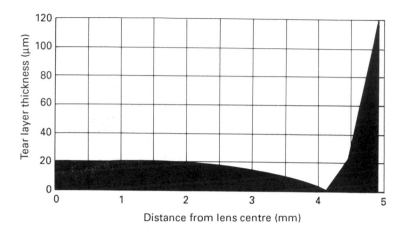

Figure 8.2 Tear layer profile/BOZD

8.5 Peripheral curves

● The first peripheral curve should be at least 0.70 mm flatter than the BOZR and rather more for lenses at the flatter end of the scale.

● For a tricurve, the final peripheral curve is typically chosen as 10.50 mm, with a width of 0.50–1.00 mm.

● A flat peripheral curve gives less corneal irritation but greater lid sensation.

● Compared with PMMA, less peripheral clearance is both feasible and desirable. Hard lenses are fitted alignment or slightly flat, so that an excessively wide periphery is unnecessary for adequate tears and oxygen flow.

● Too little peripheral clearance, however, gives unsatisfactory tears exchange because of increased capillary attraction. It can also cause arcuate staining and lens adhesion (*see* Section 6.3).

● Excessive clearance results in an unstable fitting because of an inverted tears meniscus and reduced lens adhesion (*see* Section 6.3). It can also cause peripheral dimpling and 3 and 9 o'clock staining.

Examples:

Tight periphery   7.90:8.00/8.60:8.60/9.15:9.20 (Figure 8.3)
AEL = 0.05 mm

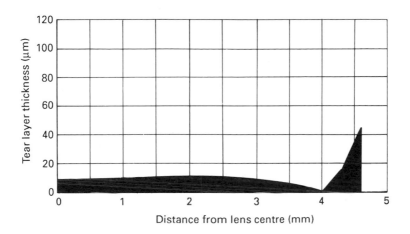

Figure 8.3 Tear layer profile/tight periphery

Average periphery   7.90:8.00/9.10:8.60/12.30:9.20 (Figure 8.4)
AEL = 0.12 mm

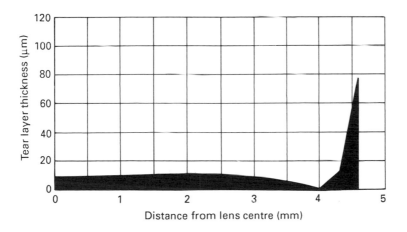

Figure 8.4 Tear layer profile/average periphery

Loose periphery   7.90:7.00/8.85:7.80/10.40:8.60/11.50:9.00
                   AEL = 0.15 mm (Figure 8.5)

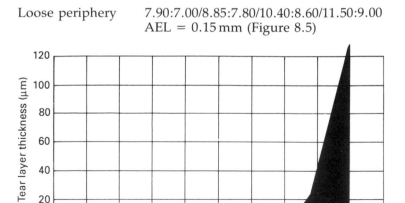

Figure 8.5 Tear layer profile/loose periphery

8.6 Back vertex power (BVP) and over-refraction

● Trial lenses should be as near as possible to the anticipated
  BVP. Minus trial lenses for hypermetropes should be avoided
  and vice versa.

● If a lens is fitted *steeper* than 'K', a *positive* liquid lens is
  created, requiring more negative power in the over-refraction
  (Figure 8.6a).

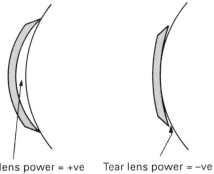

Tear lens power = +ve   Tear lens power = −ve

        (a)   (b)

Figure 8.6 (a) Steep contact lens – positive lens power; (b) flat contact lens –
negative lens power

- If a lens is fitted *flatter* than 'K', a *negative* liquid lens is created, requiring more positive power in the over-refraction (Figure 8.6b).
- Different BVPs are likely for the same degree of with- and against-the-rule astigmatism.
- The final BVP should correlate with the spectacle *Rx* after taking into account the vertex distance.

Examples: Spectacle *Rx*: −3.00 DS   K': 8.00 mm @ 180
                                                                  7.95 mm @ 90

(1) BOZR   8.10 mm   over-refraction = −0.50 D
       Trial lens −2.00 D   liquid lens   = −0.50 D
                                            final BVP   = −2.50 D

(2) BOZR   8.00 mm   over-refraction = −1.00 D
       Trial lens −2.00 D   liquid lens   =   plano
                                            final BVP   = −3.00 D

(3) BOZR   7.90 mm   over-refraction = −1.50 D
       Trial lens −2.00 D   liquid lens   = +0.50 D
                                            final BVP   = −3.50 D

Rule of thumb

A change in radius of 0.05 mm ≡ 0.25 D change in power (if the radius is in the region of 7.80 mm).

General advice

- As right and left eyes nearly always require the same TD, use different diameter trial lenses in each eye to observe two fittings at the same time.
- Use a similar technique to evaluate two BOZRs at the same time, as they do not often differ by more than 0.05 mm for similar 'K' readings.
- Check that the BVP from over-refraction correlates with the spectacle *Rx* and astigmatism after allowing for vertex distance. Repeat with a different trial lens in case of doubt.
- Do not over-refract hypermetropes with minus trial lenses and vice versa. The results are nearly always unreliable.

- If the patient was previously a PMMA wearer, order the lenses 0.02 mm thicker than normal to reduce the risk of breakage with more modern materials.

Practical advice

Hard lenses give best vision if:

- The BOZD is relatively large (>7.80 mm).
- The TD is relatively large (>9.60 mm).
- The periphery is not too wide (<1.00 mm).
- The periphery is not too flat (AEL <0.14 mm).
- Centre thickness is 0.14 mm or greater.
- Fitting is on or near flattest 'K'.

Reference

1. Stone, J. and Collins, C. (1984) Flexure of gas permeable lenses on toroidal corneas. *Optician*, **188**(4951), 8–10

Chapter 9

Fluorescein patterns and fitting

9.1 Use of fluorescein

9.1.1 Instillation of fluorescein

- A fluorescein strip is moistened with saline and excess removed by shaking.
- The patient is asked to look down while the upper lid is lifted and the wet strip gently touched onto the conjunctiva above the superior limbus, taking care not to instil excess.
- Fluorescein flows beneath the lens with the tears after two or three blinks.
- If a minim of 2% fluorescein is used, one drop only is applied with a glass rod. Some of it is allowed to wash away before inspecting the fit.

Practical advice

- *Never* use tap water to wet fluorescein strips. *Pseudomonas aeruginosa* has a strong affinity for fluorescein and may be present together with other micro-organisms such as *Acanthamoeba*.
- Do not apply the strips dry, as they can be very uncomfortable.
- It is usually more comfortable for the patient to look down to reduce lid sensation, especially with an unadapted patient.
- Sometimes, however, with very tight lids and squeamish patients it is better applied in the lower outer canthus, gently pulling down the bottom lid and resting the paper flat against the lower palpebral conjunctiva.
- Insertion of the contact lens with a viscous wetting solution may encourage the fluorescein to spread across the front surface of the lens and mask the posterior fluorescein pattern. Either use saline or give the lens longer to settle.

- Do not paint the wet strip over the conjunctiva, since too much fluorescein masks the true pattern. The excess can also stain skin and clothes.
- *Never* re-use strips with another patient because of the risk of cross-infection. Discard after use to avoid error. Use a different strip for each eye if infection is suspected.
- If a strip is re-used for the same patient, fold it as shown in Figure 9.1 to avoid contaminating the tip.

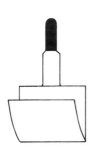

Figure 9.1 Folded fluorescein strip

9.1.2 Ultraviolet inhibitors

Some materials contain ultraviolet (UV) inhibitors, so that the fluorescein pattern with the Burton lamp shows an apparently black lens with an almost imperceptible green annulus at the periphery.

Additional fluorescein does not change the appearance and it is necessary to use the slit lamp with a blue filter to give a meaningful picture.

9.2 Examination technique

9.2.1 Burton lamp

Blue light

The essential principles in observing fluorescein patterns are:

- The method gives a dynamic assessment of lens fitting.
- Dark blue represents corneal touch.
- Green represents corneal clearance.
- Compared with slit lamp observation, the patient is more relaxed with the Burton lamp, so that both head and eyelids maintain a normal position.
- The Burton lamp uses a UV filter.

Practical advice

- Exercise care with nervous patients. They sometimes feel faint and the UV lamp is often the trigger mechanism. If in doubt, delay fluorescein examination until they are more at ease.
- Despite this, they nearly always make very good contact lens wearers.

White light

White light with low magnification allows initial investigation of lens position and movement prior to fluorescein assessment, but care is required with a photophobic patient.

9.2.2 Slit lamp

- The cobalt blue filter of the slit lamp permits evaluation of the fluorescein pattern with relatively low magnification ($\times 6$ to $\times 10$).
- A wide beam of 3–5 mm is used for general assessment.
- A narrow slit beam with higher magnification gives a qualitative indication of tear layer thickness and corneal clearance.
- The head and lids are not in a relaxed position on the instrument, so that the assessment of lens centration is not completely reliable.
- The fluorescein pattern appears normal even if the lens material contains a UV inhibitor.

9.3 Fitting

- The central and peripheral fit are independent variables and should always be assessed separately.
- The fitting should be evaluated with the lens both centred on the apex of the cornea and in a decentred position.
- Lens movement during and after a blink should be noted.
- Lens position after a blink is important.
- Lens movement on eye excursions is also significant.

9.4 Correct fitting

9.4.1 Assessment with white light

Excursion lag

With the lids in a normal position, the lens periphery should not extend beyond the limbal area even with wide excursions of the eye.

Static lag

If the lids are held apart and the lens pushed upwards, it should drop slowly of its own accord.

9.4.2 Assessment with fluorescein

ALIGNMENT FITTING (e.g. with modern multicurve designs)

Appearance

The ideal fluorescein pattern should show three fitting areas (Figure 9.2):

- Alignment or the merest hint of apical clearance over the central 7.00 mm.

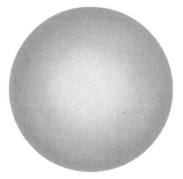

Figure 9.2 Alignment fitting

- Mid-peripheral alignment over about 1.50 mm.
- Edge clearance about 0.5 mm wide.

APICALLY CLEAR FITTING (e.g. with PMMA)

Appearance

- Fluorescein pooling over the central 5.00 mm.

- Mid-peripheral alignment.
- Edge clearance about 1.00 wide.

FLATTER THAN 'K' FITTING (e.g. most aspherics)

Appearance

- Alignment or light touch over the central 5.00 mm.
- Mid-peripheral alignment.
- Narrow edge clearance just under 0.5 mm wide.

9.5 Flat fittings

Appearance (Figure 9.3a and b)

- The fitting pattern gives a dense central area of dark blue touch surrounded by fluorescein to the edge of the lens.

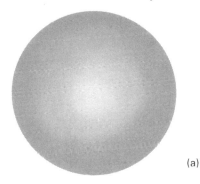

(a)

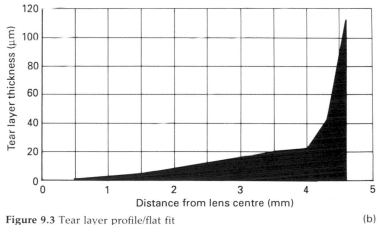

Figure 9.3 Tear layer profile/flat fit   (b)

- The area of touch is small with an indistinct as opposed to sharply demarcated border.

- Fluorescein encroaches beneath the periphery of the central portion where alignment would be expected with a correct fit.

- The lens is unstable and decentres.

- If the lens drops, it may show inferior fluorescein pooling. This is not an indication of steepness, since the lens is overhanging the lower peripheral cornea. If it is repositioned, central touch is observed.

- The entire periphery of the lens shows clearance as a wide area of fluorescein.

- Blinking gives excessive and rapid lens movement which may well be uncomfortable.

- Arcuate movement occurs when dropping between blinks or with static lag.

To correct a flat fit

- Use a steeper BOZR to improve centration.

- Increase the TD to stabilize the lens.

- Increase the BOZD to give a larger sag and steepen the fit.

- Use tighter peripheral curves to reduce dynamic forces and the effect of the lids.

- Use a thinner lens to reduce mobility.

Practical advice

- Use a steeper BOZR to give the greatest effect on the fluorescein pattern.

- All other remedies have a lesser effect and the choice of action depends on the degree of flatness.

- Carefully evaluate the TD. If the lens is already large enough, further increase might not be feasible.

- Increasing the BOZD has a greater effect on the fluorescein pattern than making the lens larger.

- Use tighter or narrower peripheries to help the lens centre better.

- All modifications to an existing lens tend to loosen the fit. A flat fitting almost invariably requires a new lens

---

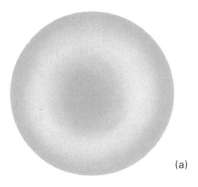

(a)

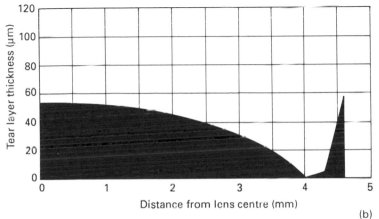

Distance from lens centre (mm)

(b)

Figure 9.4 Tear layer profile/steep fit

9.6 Steep fittings

Appearance (Figures 9.4a and b)

- The fluorescein pattern gives central pooling.
- An air bubble is sometimes present with excessive central clearance.
- Heavy bearing is seen at the transition as an area of dark blue touch beyond the central pooling.
- The smaller the area of central pooling, the greater the degree of steepness.
- The periphery gives only a thin annulus of fluorescein around the lens edge.
- There is little lens movement on blinking.

To correct a steep fit

- Use a flatter BOZR.
- Decrease the TD to increase lens mobility.
- Decrease the BOZD to give a smaller sag.
- Use flatter peripheral curves to increase the dynamic forces on the lens.
- Use a thicker lens.
- Fenestrate (*see* Section 24.3).

Practical advice

- Use a flatter BOZR to give the greatest effect on the fluorescein pattern.
- Carefully evaluate corneal and pupil sizes before reducing the TD and BOZD.
- Central fenestration is generally a last resort, but encourages tear flow beneath the lens apex and increases mobility.
- All modifications tend to loosen the fit. Several adjustments can therefore be made to improve an existing steep lens.

Clinical equivalents (*see* Section 15.1)

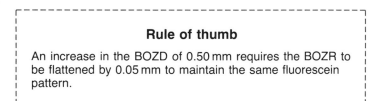

Rule of thumb

An increase in the BOZD of 0.50 mm requires the BOZR to be flattened by 0.05 mm to maintain the same fluorescein pattern.

Example 1: 7.70:7.00 ≡ 7.75:7.50 ≡ 7.80:8.00

The principle of clinical equivalents still applies to an elliptical cornea, but the differences found with tear layer theory are greater [1].

Example 2: 7.70:7.00 = 7.75:7.70 = 7.80:8.50

Rule of thumb

An increase in the BOZD of 0.70 mm requires an increase in the BOZR of 0.05 mm to give the same tear layer thickness.

9.7 Peripheral fitting

The ideal peripheral clearance is 60–80 μm – equivalent to an edge lift of 0.12–0.15 mm. It depends on corneal topography and method of fitting. In practical terms, this gives an annulus of fluorescein about 0.50 mm wide at the edge of the lens. The limit of clinical significance is about 10 μm [2].

TIGHT PERIPHERY

Appearance

● Good centration.

● Periphery presses the limbus on blinking and may cause discomfort.

● Poor tears exchange under the lens and several blinks necessary for fluorescein circulation.

To improve a tight periphery

An increase in edge clearance of at least 10–15 μm is necessary to give a discernible change in fluorescein pattern. Axial edge lift should be increased in increments of 0.03 mm (e.g. from 0.12 mm to 0.15 mm).

● Use a flatter peripheral radius (e.g. 10.75 mm instead of 10.25 mm).

● Add one or more flatter peripheral curves (e.g. 12.25 mm, 0.4 mm wide; or 15.00 mm, 0.2 mm wide).

● Increase the width of the peripheral curves.

● Use a flatter BOZR and smaller BOZD.

● Increase blending of peripheral curves.

● Change the lens design. Centration affects the peripheral interaction with the cornea.

LOOSE PERIPHERY

Appearance

- Lens rides high and does not drop after a blink.
- Bubbles are found at the edge and superior dimpling may occur.
- The edge lifts away from the cornea on blinking.
- The lens is unstable on excursion movements.
- Frequently gives 3 and 9 o'clock staining.

To improve a loose periphery

To improve a loose periphery requires a decrease in edge clearance of at least 10–15 μm. The axial edge lift is decreased in increments of 0.03 mm (e.g. from 0.15 mm to 0.12 mm).

- Use a tighter peripheral radius (e.g. 10.00 mm instead of 10.50 mm).
- Reduce the width of the peripheral curves.
- Use a larger BOZD, possibly with a flatter BOZR to compensate.
- Change the lens design and possibly try an aspheric.

General advice

- Use a negative carrier for low riding plus lenses.
- Aspheric lenses sometimes give better centration and comfort with plus lenses.
- A displaced corneal apex causes lens decentration even if the fitting is not too flat. Use a larger TD if flare is a problem.
- Tight lids with a toric cornea also cause decentration. Consider a back surface toric lens.

References

1. Atkinson, T. (1987) The development of the back surface design of rigid lenses. *Contax*, Nov., 5–18
2. Atkinson, T. (1985) A computer assisted and clinical assessment of current trends in gas permeable lens design. *Optician*, **189**(4976), 16–22

Chapter 10

Aspheric lenses

Aspheric lens design has evolved because clinical models have shown the overall form of the cornea to be elliptical [1–3]. The variation in the shape of an ellipse is called the eccentricity (e) and is an important factor in lens design and fitting. Mathematically, it is always less than 1 (*see* Section 7.4).

10.1 Advantages and disadvantages of aspherics

ADVANTAGES OF ASPHERICS

● Fit more closely to the corneal topography (Figure 10.1).

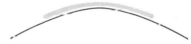

Figure 10.1 Aspheric lens showing close fit to corneal topography

● Distribute pressure more evenly over the cornea.
● Edge lift or 'Z' value is smaller, giving less lid sensation.
● Can sometimes fit up to 4.00 D of astigmatism.
● Some designs can give improved distance vision, others can assist presbyopia (*see* Section 23.4.2).
● Absence of transition zones assists tear flow.

DISADVANTAGES OF ASPHERICS

● Manufacture requires sophisticated lathes.
● Reproducibility and verification more difficult.
● Aberrations with some back surface designs.
● Decentration if fitted flatter than 'K' to obtain movement.
● Decentration with a decentred corneal apex.

10.2 Aspheric designs

10.2.1 Fully aspheric lenses

A completely aspheric back surface causes problems where the lens edge presses into the peripheral cornea. A small, spherical bevel is therefore usually incorporated into the design (*see* Section 10.2.2).

Bi-aspheric designs are available which have a posterior central optic zone with an eccentricity of 0.4–0.45 aligning over the central 7 mm of the cornea. The peripheral zone is hyperbolic to give an edge clearance of 8–10 μm.

10.2.2 Mainly aspheric/part sphere

These designs consist of a mainly aspheric back surface with a spherical peripheral curve. The spherical curve is needed to prevent the elliptical edge from pressing into the cornea. It also assists tears exchange and lens removal.

Two common designs are the Persecon E (Ciba) and Hydron GP 20/50.

Persecon E

The Persecon E has an eccentricity of $e = 0.4$ and rate of flattening $p = 0.84$. It has a spherical periphery between 10 mm and 12 mm in radius and between 0.20 mm and 0.30 mm wide, to give an edge clearance of 20–60 μm.

GP 20/50

The GP 20/50 does not have a fixed eccentricity and is therefore considered a 'multi-aspheric' or 'differential flattening aspheric' [4] with an eccentricity of $e = 0.56$. It has a spherical edge band about 11.50 mm in radius and 0.25 mm wide. This offers a choice of periphery that gradually increases in tear thickness beyond the central 6 mm to either 29 or 39 μm. The numerical suffix relates to the *Dk* of the material.

10.2.3 Mainly spherical/part asphere

These consist of a central spherical portion with an aspheric peripheral zone area and are termed 'polynomial aspheric designs'. The aspheric zone is, in turn, surrounded by a small spherical edge bevel.

Quantum

The Quantum lens (Bausch and Lomb) has a 3.50–4.00 mm central spherical portion with an aspheric periphery. The edge has a radius of 11.25 mm, 0.3 mm wide [5].

10.3 Principles of fitting

10.3.1 Fully aspheric lenses

Bi-aspheric designs are generally fitted on or slightly flatter than 'K' (e.g. Hanita). With toric corneas, the central radius is selected in relation to mean 'K'.

The fluorescein pattern should show the central and mid-peripheral alignment of a uniform tear layer, with the lens edge giving a well-defined tears meniscus. The lens position should be central or high riding, but not crossing the superior limbus.

With toric corneas, the typical band of central touch is acceptable. Mid-peripheral bearing indicates the need for a flatter or smaller lens, whereas hard central touch or decentration requires a steeper fitting.

The bi-aspheric nature of the lens design gives good edge clearance and tears exchange. Residual astigmatism, however, may be induced by lens decentration because of the differential power effect of the sagittal and tangential radii towards the lens periphery.

10.3.2 Mainly aspheric/part sphere

Persecon E

The Persecon E design can be manufactured from either CAB or silicone acrylate (*see* Section 5.1). In both cases it is fitted slightly flatter than flattest 'K'. The total diameter is chosen according to corneal size: 8.80 mm or 9.30 mm for corneas up to 11.0 mm, and 9.80 mm or 10.30 mm for those larger than 11.0 mm.

A correct fitting shows alignment or the suggestion of light central touch. In case of decentration, a larger lens should be tried before steepening the curvature. The edge bevel is cut with a common tangent to the ellipse to give good comfort.

GP 20/50

The GP 20/50 tends to be more stable when fitted slightly steeper than alignment, showing a trace of central fluorescein. Excessive edge clearance should be avoided or the fitting becomes unstable [5]. Diameters available are 9.20 mm and 9.80 mm and are selected according to corneal size.

Examples: 'K' 7.89 mm × 7.83 mm
Persecon E: 8.00:9.30
GP 20:   7.90:9.20 (Figures 10.2 and 10.3)

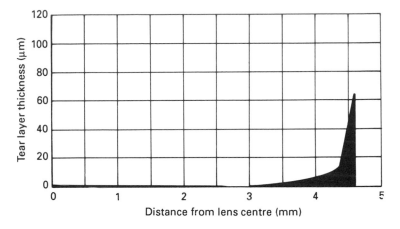

Figure 10.2 Tear layer profile/GP20 (7.89 meridian)

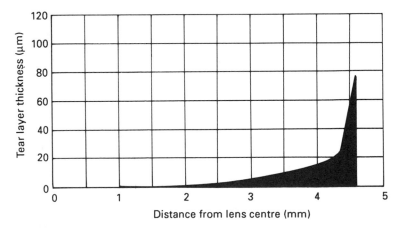

Figure 10.3 Tear layer profile/GP20 (7.83 meridian)

10.3.3 Mainly spherical/part asphere

Quantum

The spherical central radius is selected 0.10 mm steeper than flattest 'K' to allow the aspheric mid-peripheral portion to align with the cornea. The fluorescein pattern gives slight central pooling surrounded by an area of alignment with peripheral edge clearance. The lens design can give excessive edge clearance with steep corneas and too little clearance with flat corneas. Quantum does not ride as high as some of the flatter fitting designs and is useful where it is desirable to avoid lid attachment. The usual total diameter is 9.60 mm. To help centration 10.20 mm lenses are available, but even 9.60 mm is too large for some small corneas. Only plus lenses are available in a 9.00 mm diameter.

10.3.4 General fitting considerations

Aspheric lenses:

- Do not require such critical fitting because fewer parameters.
- Need to be fitted slightly flat to give adequate movement and sufficient edge clearance (except designs like Quantum).
- Flat fitting, however, tends to give decentration as a common problem.

Spherical cornea

The ideal fit is alignment or slightly flatter than alignment. A slightly flat fit gives light central touch, but because of even pressure distribution any stress to the cornea is kept to a minimum.

A flat fit shows hard central touch surrounded by an excessive annulus of fluorescein. There is increased lid sensation and unstable vision.

A steep fit gives excessive central pooling with a sharp border, surrounded by a peripheral ring of hard touch and a very narrow meniscus of fluorescein at the periphery.

Toric cornea

The ideal fit is also alignment or slightly flatter than flattest 'K' to minimize lens flexure and maintain good acuity.

Practical advice

The axial edge lift of an aspheric lens is less than with the equivalent multicurve. It is sometimes possible to fit higher degrees of astigmatism because of the reduced edge stand-off in the steeper meridian.

10.4 Fluorescein patterns compared with spherical lenses

● A much more gradual change in the fluorescein pattern from centre to periphery.

● True alignment can be achieved if the correct eccentricity has been assessed (e.g. with a topographic keratometer [6]).

● The peripheral tear layer thickness increases more gradually towards the edge.

● Larger lenses have to be used to help centration.

References

1. Bibby, M. (1976) Computer assisted photokeratoscopy and contact lens design. *Optician*, **171**(4423), 37–43; **171**(4424), 11–17; **171**(4425), 15–17
2. Kiely, P.M., Smith, G. and Carney, L.C. (1984) Meridional variations in corneal shape. *American Journal of Optometry and Physiological Optics*, **61**, 619–626
3. Guillon, M., Lydon, D.P.M. and Wilson, C. (1986) Corneal topography: a clinical model. *Ophthalmic and Physiological Optics*, **6**, 47–56
4. Bennett, A.G. (1988) Aspherical and continuous curve contact lenses, part IV. *Optometry Today*, **28**, 433–444
5. Atkinson, T.C.O. (1989) Towards a new gas permeable lens geometry. *Optician*, **197**(5181), 13–17
6. Rabbetts, R.B. (1985) The Humphrey auto keratometer. *Ophthalmic and Physiological Optics*, **5**, 451–458

Chapter 11

Lens specification and verification

11.1 British and International Standards

British Standard BS 3521: Part 3: 1987 *Glossary of Terms and Symbols* is a dual publication of International Standard ISO 8320 – 1986.

BS 5750 covers manufacturers of assessed capability and implies that verification, production, tolerances, quality assurance, and sampling conform to this standard.

11.1.1 British Standard terms

The terminology for a standard tricurve lens in British Standard symbols is:

$$r_0 \; : \; \varnothing_0 \; / \; r_1 \; : \; \varnothing_1 \; / \; r_2 \; : \; \varnothing_r \quad t_c \quad \text{BVP} \quad \text{Tint}$$
$$\text{BOZR} : \text{BOZD} / \text{BPZR}_1 : \text{BPZD}_1 / \text{BPZR}_2 : \text{TD}$$

Example

7.90:7.80/8.70:8.60/10.75:9.20 t_c 0.15 BVP −3.00D Tint light blue

7.90 = back optic zone radius (BOZR) r_0
7.80 = back optic zone diameter (BOZD) $\varnothing_0$
8.70 = first back peripheral radius r_1
8.60 = first back peripheral zone diameter $\varnothing_1$
10.75 = second back peripheral radius r_2
9.20 = total diameter $\varnothing_T$
0.15 = geometric centre thickness t_c
−3.00 = back vertex power (BVP)

For a lenticular lens (reduced optic):

7.90:7.80/8.70:8.60/10.75:9.20 t_c 0.45 t_e 0.16 BVP +10.00 D
FOZD 8.30 Tint light blue

0.45 = geometric centre thickness t_c
0.16 = edge thickness t_e

+10.00 = back vertex power (BVP)
  8.30 = front optic zone diameter $\emptyset_{a0}$

The subscript 'a' indicates an anterior surface component and the format is the same for both plus and minus lenses.

11.2 Examples of hard lens types and fittings

(Assuming a spherical 'K' reading of 7.75 mm and low minus power)

INDIVIDUAL DESIGNS

- TD 8.60 mm   CAEL 0.12 mm [1]
  7.80:7.00/9.00:7.80/10.90:8.60
- TD 9.00 mm   CAEL 0.15 mm [1]
  7.80:7.00/8.75:7.80/10.10:8.60/11.30:9.00
- TD 9.20 mm   CAEL 0.12 mm [2]
  7.80:8.00/8.80:8.60/12.30:9.20
- Atkinson high Dk design [3]   TLT 13 μm, EC 60 μm
  7.80:7.70/8.30:8.20/9.20:9.20
- TD 9.50 mm   CAEL 0.175 mm [4]
  7.80:7.50/8.90:8.50/10.00:9.00/11.15:9.50
- Atkinson high Dk design [3]   TLT 12 μm, EC 60 μm
  7.80:8.30/8.20:8.80/9.00:9.80

PROPRIETARY DESIGNS

- Mini Boston (Kelvin): 7.80:7.70/8.55:8.20/10.40:9.00
- Quantum (Bausch and Lomb): 7.70/9.60
- Persecon E (Ciba): 7.80/9.30 or 7.80/9.80
- Standard Polycon II (Pilkington Barnes-Hind): 7.80:7.80/AEL 0.10 at 9.00

11.3 Hard lens verification

All lenses should ideally be checked before use:

- To ensure the accuracy of trial lenses.

- To ensure prescription lenses are suitable for dispensing.
- To establish the specification of the patient's existing lenses.
- Where lens parameters are thought to have altered.
- Where lenses are thought to have distorted.
- To confirm that lenses are being worn in the correct eyes.
- To confirm that current and old lenses have not been mixed up.
- To ensure records contain full details of lens specification.

11.3.1 Back optic zone radius (BOZR)

RADIUSCOPE

Based on Drysdale's method which measures the distance between the lens surface and the centre of curvature.

Practical advice

- To obtain a good image, ensure the lens is well dried before being placed on a drop of distilled water in the concave holder.
- To help location of the images, ensure the instrument light is at the centre of the lens.
- Travelling from the zero to the second position the image of the bulb filament is seen. The quality of this image gives an indication of any lens distortion.
- Always take two or three readings and average the results.
- The image at the lens surface is usually much larger and brighter than that at the centre of curvature, as well as showing any surface scratches.
- The zero reading with unstable hard lenses can 'creep' and may require several attempts before giving a reliable result. If the creeping does not stop, average the first three readings.

OTHER METHODS

Keratometer

Uses a lens holder with a front surface silvered mirror. 0.03 mm is added to correct for the concave surface [5].

Radius checking device

The radius is derived from the focimeter FVP, using refractive index and thick lens formula [6].

Toposcope

Uses moire fringes [5].

11.3.2 Peripheral radius (BPZR)

Peripheral radii can be measured with the radiuscope if the lens is tilted and the band width is at least 1 mm.

A qualitative assessment can be made with a Burton lamp by observing the reflection of the white light tube in the lens surface.

11.3.3 Total diameter (TD) and zone diameters (BPZD)

Measuring magnifier (band magnifier)

Consists of an engraved graticule plus an adjustable eyepiece with ×7 magnification. The lens is repositioned on the scale for different zones, and measurement is easier with sharp transitions.

V gauge

Consists of a V-shaped channel graduated between 6.0 mm and 12.5 mm. Only measures TD.

Projection magnifier

Projects a magnified image of the entire lens onto a calibrated screen (e.g. Zeiss DL2).

Practical advice

- Ensure lens is dry or it can be difficult to remove from a smooth surface because of capillary attraction.
- Avoid wet cell instruments because of difficulty in lens manipulation.

11.3.4 Back and front vertex power (BVP and FVP)

Focimeter

- Place focimeter in a vertical position or use a V-slot holder.
- For BVP, place the concave surface towards the focimeter.
- The lens must be placed as close as possible to the focimeter, either by using a very small stop or by removing the stop cover. The reading may still give more plus or less minus than the true BVP because of the steep lens radius.
- For FVP, place the convex surface towards the focimeter stop. FVP reads less than the BVP, with a greater difference in plus powers than minus.

Practical advice

- Note the quality of the image on the focimeter. Distortion indicates a poor optic.
- A good image does not necessarily guarantee a distortion-free optic because a small stop is used and only the centre of the lens is measured.

11.3.5 Centre and edge thickness (t_c and t_e)

Thickness gauge

Consists of a spring-loaded, ball-ended probe geared to a direct reading scale.

Practical advice

- Take several readings of the lens edge, as the thickness may vary around the circumference.
- Take care not to damage a thin edge.

Radiuscope

The lens holder is left dry and the target focused on each lens surface in turn. The distance between the two images multiplied by the refractive index of the material gives the central lens thickness.

11.3.6 Edge form

Edge form is best examined with about ×20 magnification using either a hand loupe or the slit lamp.

11.3.7 Surface quality

Surface scratches and defects can be assessed in a variety of ways:

- Projection magnifier with a clean dry lens.
- Slit lamp, using transillumination.
- Band magnifier.
- Radiuscope by examining the first image.

11.3.8 Material

Confirming lens material is difficult, although comparison of specific gravity measurements can give an approximate guide. The most reliable indication can sometimes be colour, since certain hard lenses are available in only one distinctive tint (e.g. Conflex, very pale blue; Polycon II, medium blue).

11.3.9 Other features

- Engravings (e.g. 'R' or a 'dot' for the right lens).
- Laboratory codes.
- Fenestrations – number, position, size and finish.
- Tint.
- Prism ballast – increased edge thickness at the base.
- Truncation.
- Carrier design – assessed by edge measurement.

11.4 Tolerances

See Table 11.1

Table 11.1 Suggested tolerances

Parameter	BSI/ISO suggested tolerances
BOZR	± 0.05 mm
BPZR	± 0.10 mm
BOZD	± 0.20 mm
TD	± 0.10 mm
Edge and centre thickness	± 0.02 mm
BVP	± 0.12 D up to ± 7.00 D
	± 0.25 D from ± 7.00 D to ± 14.00
	± 0.50 D over ± 14.00 D

Practical advice

- The easiest methods for practitioner verification are:

BOZR	Radiuscope
DIAMETERS	Band magnifier
POWER	Focimeter
THICKNESS	Thickness gauge
CONDITION	Projection or band magnifier

- Hard and PMMA lenses flatten on both front and back surfaces with hydration [7]. Flattening relates to BVP (greater with high minus) and centre thickness.

- New lenses should be hydrated for 24 h before a reliable measurement can be made.

- Very rapid changes in BOZR also occur on dehydration [8].

- Hard trial lenses should be kept hydrated. PMMA lenses in powers < ±10.00 D are reliable if dry.

References

1. Stone, J. (1975) Corneal lenses with constant axial edge lift. *Ophthalmic Optician*, **15**, 818–824
2. Atkinson, T.C.O. (1980) The return of hard times, part II. *Journal of the British Contact Lens Association*, **3**, 105–112
3. Atkinson, T.C.O. (1987) The development of the back surface design of rigid lenses. *Contax*, Nov., 5–18
4. Rabbetts, R.B. (1976) Large corneal lenses with constant axial edge lift. *Ophthalmic Optician*, **16**, 236–239
5. Watts, R. (1989) Hard lens verification procedures. In *Contact Lenses*, A.J. Phillips and J. Stone (eds), Butterworths, London, pp. 440–462
6. Sarver, M.D. and Kerr, K. (1964) A radius of curvature measuring device for contact lenses. *American Journal of Optometry*, **41**, 481–489

7. Phillips, A.J. (1969) Alterations in curvature of the finished corneal lens. *Ophthalmic Optician*, **9**, 980–1110
8. Pearson, R.M. (1977) Dimensional stability of several hard contact lens materials. *American Journal of Optometry and Physiological Optics*, **54**, 826–833

Chapter 12

PMMA corneal lens fitting

12.1 Physiological problems caused by PMMA

PMMA lenses have in many cases now been worn for over 30 years [1]. Patients are often quite happy with their lenses and it is only at aftercare examination that the practitioner may detect corneal changes. In other cases, patients seek advice because of reduced wearing time, red eyes or depressed vision.

The common changes found with long-term PMMA wear are:

- Epithelial oedema.
- Central punctate epithelial staining.
- Chronic 3 and 9 o'clock staining.
- Stromal oedema.
- Folds in Descemet's membrane.
- Endothelial distortion.
- Endothelial polymegathism.
- Reduced corneal sensitivity.

These changes are due to chronic lack of oxygen and drying of the corneal tissue, and the mechanical action of the lens. The combination of these long-term effects produces the loss of tolerance known as 'corneal exhaustion syndrome'.

Also found, although less commonly, are:

- Dellen.
- Opacification and vascularization in the 3 and 9 o'clock meridians.
- Vertical striae.
- Fischer–Schweitzer mosaic pattern.
- Hyperaemic lids.
- Papillary conjunctivitis (PC).

12.2 When PMMA should still be fitted

There are, however, a minority of cases where PMMA may still be considered:

● Where flexure problems with modern hard lenses give unsatisfactory acuity, especially if a thin lens is necessary.
● Where a trial lens is needed to check the fluorescein pattern of complicated fitting (e.g. keratoconus or opaque cosmetic) and PMMA is significantly cheaper.
● Children or clumsy patients who may break modern hard lenses too easily.
● Deposit problems with all other hard lens materials.
● Myopia control.
● Where an inert material is required because of allergies (e.g. PC).
● To give better surface wetting.

12.3 Fitting considerations for PMMA compared with hard lenses

● Fitted with slight apical clearance to encourage good tears exchange, whereas modern hard lenses are usually fitted in alignment.
● Edge clearance is also greater to allow good tears exchange.
● BOZD is usually smaller to cover less corneal area. Modern hard lenses have relatively large BOZDs to avoid flare.
● PMMA must be well blended to avoid oedema and arcuate staining.
● PMMA can be ultra-thin (0.01 mm or less) to avoid corneal distortion. Very thin hard lenses flex and cause visual problems.
● High minus powers in PMMA can avoid the lens distortion which occurs with some less stable hard lens materials.
● PMMA is more easily modified and polished than many hard lens materials because of their surface characteristics and brittleness.

12.4 Modern PMMA fitting

PMMA is fitted according to the following different criteria because of its impermeability:

- The BOZR is chosen 0.05–0.10 mm steeper than flattest 'K'.
- For a toric cornea, the BOZR is chosen half to two-thirds between flattest and steepest 'K'.
- TDs smaller than 9.50 mm are used for low powers; 9.20 mm is a good average diameter.
- A BOZD of approximately 7.00 mm is used for a TD of 9.20 mm, and 7.50 mm for 9.50 mm lens.
- Edges should be well rounded.
- Centre thickness should be ≥0.10 mm for dimensional stability.

Practical advice

- Give a slower wearing schedule (*see* Section 26.3).
- Laboratory instructions should always state 'very well blended', as modern hard lens blending is inadequate.
- Where it is essential to fit PMMA and oedema occurs, reduce BOZD or TD; increase edge lift or blending; fenestrate.

12.5 Orthokeratology and myopia control

Orthokeratology is a procedure designed to reduce artificially the refractive error of (usually) myopic eyes by fitting lenses increasingly flatter than 'K' in order to change progressively the corneal curvature [2,3]. It is controversial due to the lack of extensive clinical evaluation, although the procedure does seem to work in many cases. The main problem is the impermanence and poor stability of the refractive result, so that 'retainer' lenses are required for some time each day. Long-term corneal distortion is also a possibility.

It is not the same as myopia control, where conventionally fitted PMMA has been demonstrated to reduce the rate of increase of myopia over several years [4,5] (*see* Section 29.2.1).

References

1. Boyd, H. (1971) Analysis of 1,000 consecutive contact lens cases. First Scientific Congress of the European Contact Lens Society of Ophthalmologists, London, June
2. *Orthokeratology* (1972), Vol. 1, International Orthokeratology Section of NERF publication, NERF, USA
3. *Orthokeratology* (1974), Vol. 2, International Orthokeratology Section of NERF publication, NERF, USA
4. Stone, J. (1976) The possible influence of contact lenses on myopia. *British Journal of Physiological Optics*, **31**, 89–114
5. Perrigin, J. Perrigin, D. Quintero, S and Grosvenor, T. (1990) Silicone/acrylate contact lenses for myopia control: 3-year results. *Optometry and Vision Science*, **67**, 764–765

Chapter 13

Refitting PMMA wearers

Refitting long-term PMMA wearers represents one of the more difficult aspects of modern practice, especially where there are no previous details available. The procedure is further complicated because, however carefully measurement and fitting are carried out, changes are likely to occur as the cornea comes 'off the influence' of PMMA. The correct course of action in nearly all cases is to refit with modern hard lenses. It is not generally feasible to move directly from PMMA to soft lenses (*see* Section 13.2.4).

13.1 Problems of refitting

13.1.1 At initial refitting

- The cornea may show considerable signs of oedema and distortion.
- 'K' readings may be very different from the measurements when fitting has ultimately been completed.
- 'K' readings may exhibit considerable distortion.
- Accurate refraction may be very difficult if not impossible with poor retinoscopy reflex.
- Visual acuity may be depressed because of corneal oedema.
- It is frequently impossible to measure accurately the BOZR of old, distorted lenses.

13.1.2 As refitting progresses

- 'K' readings change, possibly making the initial fitting unsatisfactory. This may occur as long as 12 months later.
- The degree of corneal astigmatism alters.
- The BVP often requires more minus power after 1–3 weeks.
- Patients may experience greater difficulty with foreign bodies

as well as greater lens awareness when corneal sensitivity recovers.

13.2 Refitting procedures

13.2.1 General points

- Patients should understand the possible difficulties and that refitting requires careful follow-up.
- Patients should come for their appointment wearing the existing PMMA lenses, as with spectacle prescribing (*see* Section 28.4).
- If they exist, old pre-contact lens spectacles should be examined. They are unlikely to be accurate, but offer clues to the type of ametropia and degree of astigmatism.
- Measure the old lenses where possible.

13.2.2 Refitting with hard lenses

Fitting

- The slit lamp is used to observe the extent of any corneal oedema or lens-induced staining.
- The PMMA lenses are assessed with white light and fluorescein, noting where improvements to the physical fitting may be made.
- The PMMA lenses are removed and measured.
- 'K' readings are taken as carefully as possible, but they may be unreliably flat and show an artificial degree of astigmatism.
- An assessment of the refraction is made.
- The initial trial lenses are based on 'K' readings, but measurements of old lenses are taken into account. Much more reliance is placed on the fluorescein appearance than 'K's, although this is also difficult because central oedema may give a conus-like fitting.

Choice of design

- Hard lenses give better vision if steep fittings are avoided.
- PMMA difficulties such as poor centration or flare can often be solved by fitting a larger optic and total diameter.

- There is less 3 and 9 o'clock staining with narrower edge lifts.

- For patients with very tight lids, designs are avoided with narrow edge lift, especially aspherics. There is an increased chance of lens adhesion.

- If both practitioner and patient are perfectly happy with the existing PMMA design, it can be duplicated in a modern hard lens material.

Choice of material

- A low to medium Dk material can be used if the patient is asymptomatic and there are no particular signs of oedema.

- A medium to high Dk should be considered where there are more obvious corneal changes.

- Use moulded CAB where there is predisposition to 3 and 9 o'clock staining.

- Use fluorosilicone acrylates or CAB, and avoid silicone acrylates, where protein deposits are likely to be a problem (e.g. hay fever sufferers, vernal catarrh).

- Avoid CAB and other less rigid materials with tight lids and toric corneas, since lenses may flex or distort.

- Avoid CAB and other easily scratched materials with patients prone to surface damage.

- Avoid brittle materials for initial refitting. Patients used to handling relatively robust PMMA are likely to have breakage problems.

Ordering lenses

- More confidence can be placed on the final fitting if it correlates with 'K' readings, old lens measurements, refraction or calculated lens BVP.

- Refraction frequently shows an increase in minus of 0.25–0.50 D after about 2 weeks. Myopes should therefore be fully corrected and binocular adds are not usually given. Take into account the BVP of the old lenses and possibly even over-correct by -0.25 D.

- Carefully specify centre and edge thickness where possible.

Practical advice

- Use a laboratory where lenses can be returned for exchange, modification or credit.
- Fees should take into account the extra time and lens costs which may be required in refitting PMMA.

Follow-up

- The first check-up should be after about 2 weeks to reassess the fitting, corneas and lens powers.
- Reconsider the lens material.
- Unless there is a gross change in fitting or power, lenses should not be modified for another 4–6 weeks. By this time, most corneal changes will have stabilized and a spectacle *Rx* may also be feasible.
- In some cases, further minor changes may be found up to 12 months later.

Problems

A minority of patients cannot adapt to modern hard lenses because of:

- Physical discomfort, relating to surface wetting properties and increased corneal sensitivity.
- Poor visual acuity, relating to lens flexure or distortion.
- Deposits and greasing problems.
- PC.

If these problems cannot be resolved, the practitioner may be obliged to return to an improved design of PMMA or change to soft lenses after a further 6–8 weeks.

Patient advice

Patients should be carefully advised on lens collection about:

- The importance of using the recommended solutions and enzyme tablets where necessary.
- The shorter life span compared with PMMA.
- The increased risk of scratching and breakage.

- To note any lens adherence.
- Increased discomfort with foreign bodies.

13.2.3 Refitting with soft lenses

Except for very special circumstances, it is not generally feasible to refit PMMA wearers directly with soft lenses.

- The problems listed at initial fitting and as fitting progresses are much more significant with soft lenses.
- As the 'K' readings change, the degree of astigmatism may alter in an unpredictable fashion. Initially good acuity may deteriorate as corneal toricity changes.
- Some PMMA wearers find the gelatinous feel of a soft lens quite unpleasant on the eye.
- Many PMMA wearers have solutions difficulties, both with allergic responses and the additional complexities of soft lens disinfection.

Practical advice

- Do not refit PMMA directly with soft.
- However, where it is essential to provide PMMA wearers with soft lenses, it is generally better to refit first with hard lenses as an intermediate step. After about 6–8 weeks, the cornea and refraction may have stabilized sufficiently to make soft lens fitting feasible.
- Disposable lenses have a place in coping with a continuously altering corneal curvature and refraction.

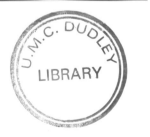

Chapter 14

Scleral lens fitting

14.1 When scleral lenses should still be fitted

ADVANTAGES OF SCLERAL LENSES

- Almost never lost because they are held in place by the eyelids; capillary attraction is to the sclera rather than the cornea.
- Robust and dimensionally stable.
- Do not deteriorate.
- Can be handled by less dextrous patients (e.g. aphakics).
- Dry storage is preferred with PMMA.
- Less expensive to maintain.
- Lid sensation is much less than with corneal lenses.
- Foreign bodies are uncommon except on insertion.

INDICATIONS

Therapeutic for irregular eyes

- High astigmatism.
- Advanced keratoconus.
- Corneal grafts.
- Traumatized eyes.
- Microphthalmos.
- Cosmetic cases.

Therapeutic for protection

The large size of a scleral lens protects the anterior eye and enables the retention of a tears reservoir in abnormal conditions.

- Corneal exposure.

- Dry eyes.
- Trichiasis.

Other applications

- Ptosis.
- Centration difficulties with high-power corneal lenses.
- Intermittent use where short-term adaptation may be easier than with corneal lenses (e.g. sports).
- Dusty environment.
- Water sports.

14.2 Preformed lenses

14.2.1 Preformed designs

A preformed scleral lens is fitted without taking a mould of the eye from trial sets of predetermined shape (Figure 14.1).

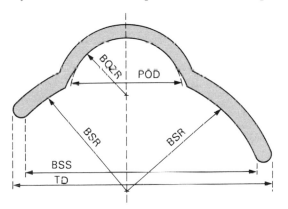

Figure 14.1 Preformed scleral lens (BOZR, back optic zone radius; POD, primary optic diameter; BSR, back scleral radius; BSS, back scleral size; TD, total diameter) (from Philips and Stone, *Contact Lenses*, 3rd edn, Butterworth-Heinemann, by permission)

Conical lenses

Developed by Feinbloom in 1936 [1]. The design consists of a spherical optic portion (BOZR), a scleral zone (BSR) of which the major part is conical, and a crescent on the temporal side which has a spherical curve.

Wide angle lenses

Introduced by Nissel in 1947 [2]. The design is a combination of spherical optic and scleral portions with a conical transition. Trial sets are extensive because they require sufficient variables for the fitting of both major parts of the lens. Examples:

BSR 12.50 mm; BOZR 8.00 mm, 8.25 mm, 8.50 mm
BSR 13.50 mm; BOZR 8.00 mm, 8.25 mm, 8.50 mm, 8.75 mm, 9.00 mm

Spherical preformed lenses

Redesigned in their present form by Bier in 1948 [3]. Lenses have a spherical optic and back scleral surface. The transition is 2.00 mm wide, with a spherical radius of curvature the mean of the back optic and scleral zone. The fit of the optic portion is established independently, using a fenestrated lens for optic measurement (FLOM). Example:

BSS 22.50 mm; BSR 12.50 mm, 13.00 mm, 13.50 mm, 14.00 mm
BSS 24.00 mm; BSR 13.00 mm, 13.50 mm, 14.00 mm, 14.50 mm

14.2.2 Modern preformed fitting

Various trial sets are used and there are two possible approaches:

● Separate fitting of the scleral and optic portions.
● Fitting both parts at the same time.

INDEPENDENT OPTIC AND SCLERAL FITTING

It is important that the scleral portion does not interfere with the optic fitting and vice versa, but the method gives good control over the independent portions. The disadvantage is that the practitioner never sees the complete and final fitting until the lens is dispensed.

Scleral portion

Trial sets vary both in back scleral radius (BSR) and back scleral size (BSS). A full set consists of 12 lenses in steps of 0.50 mm for radius and diameter, but a useful minimum range is:

Back scleral size: 22.50 mm and 24.50 mm
Back scleral radius: 12.50 mm and 14.50 mm

With experience, it is possible to judge by how much to alter the size without necessarily inspecting a second lens in situ. This does not apply to the radius where it is essential to observe the next lens [4].

Rule of thumb

If the back scleral size is increased by 1.00–1.50 mm, the back scleral radius must be flattened by 0.25 mm to give the same fitting appearance [4].

Practical advice

- Aim for a minimum clearance fitting.
- The optic radius should be no flatter than 7.50 mm at a chord width of 12.50 mm to ensure that the optic portion is clear of the cornea at all times during fitting.
- An optimum fitting scleral radius does not blanch the conjunctival blood vessels.
- A steep scleral fit bears excessively on the peripheral sclera and constricts the vessels in that area.
- A flat radius constricts the vessels around the limbus.
- The horizontal sclera is asymmetrical. It is not always possible to eliminate blanching completely so that a 75% 'glove fit' is acceptable.
- Avoid constricting the limbus wherever possible.
- Localized modification by 'grind-out' is possible.

The optic zone

The cornea is fitted using FLOM lenses, first described by Bier in 1948 [5]. They consist of an optic portion with a narrow scleral rim approximately 2 mm wide, and usually have a 13.00 mm radius. This is flatter than the limbal region it covers so that it does not interfere with the corneal fit. To assist fitting, the transition is deliberately left sharp. This can cause discomfort, so topical anaesthetic may be used. The lenses are identified by the back optic zone radius and optic zone diameter. Most lenses are optically worked to enable refraction when the correct corneal fitting has been found. Lenses have a large, 1.50 mm, peripheral fenestration and the front transition is smooth. The normal range of parameters is:

Radius: 8.00–9.50 mm in 0.25 mm steps
Diameter: 13.00–14.75 mm in 0.25 mm steps

The fitting is assessed with fluorescein and is varied by altering either the radius or diameter. The optimum fit gives clearance over the whole cornea, extending 2–3 mm beyond the limbus. A crescent-shaped air bubble should remain at the limbus (Figure 14.2).

Figure 14.2 Crescent-shaped air bubble in FLOM lens fitting

Clinical equivalents

Two lenses giving identical fitting characteristics of apical clearance with different but related parameters are known as clinical equivalents.

Rule of thumb

If the radius is flattened by 0.25 mm, the diameter must be increased by 0.50 mm to give the same apical clearance.

Example: 8.00/13.00 ≡ 8.25/13.50

SIMULTANEOUS OPTIC AND SCLERAL FITTING

The main advantage of simultaneous fitting is that the trial lens appears very close to final lens. It also avoids the discomfort of a FLOM lens and topical anaesthesia is unnecessary. However, a very large trial set is required for optimum fitting, since four variables must be considered with this system:

- Optic radius.
- Optic diameter.
- Scleral radius.
- Overall diameter.

Generally, smaller lenses and optic diameters suit steeper eyes and vice versa.

Preformed fitting is ideally carried out with a combination of simultaneous and separate systems.

14.3 Moulded (impression) fitting

Fitting sclerals from eye impressions is much better for dealing with irregular anterior ocular topography. The impression gives the negative shape of the cornea from which the scleral lens is made [6].

14.3.1 Impression materials

Alginates

- Usually Kromopan (the recommended material).
- The normal mixture is 2 g to 7 ml water, but may vary up to 5 g to 5 ml.
- Setting is faster with a higher temperature where more water may be used.

Vinyl polysiloxanes

Panasil, consisting of a base paste and hardener, is the usual choice. It does not dehydrate because no water is used and it keeps indefinitely.

14.3.2 Moulding procedure

- The eye must be anaesthetized with at least three drops of Benoxinate, one instilled from above the cornea.
- One drop instilled in the alternate eye inhibits the blink reflex.

- The eye to be moulded should look slightly down and in from the primary position. This can be achieved by dissociating the two eyes and marking on the lower lid of the alternate eye the position of the cornea which allows the eye being moulded to take up the correct position.
- The moulding shell or tray is chosen as (a) small, medium or large; and (b) left or right, since nasal and temporal sizes are different (Figure 14.3).

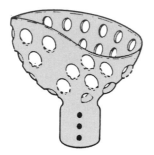

Figure 14.3 Moulding tray. The trays are colour coded (red = right; blue = left) and a system of dots denotes the size (3 dots = large; 2 dots = medium; 1 dot = small)

- The impression material is mixed and spatulated to eliminate air bubbles.
- The average setting time of the impression material is about 1 min at normal room temperature.

Injection method

- More time is available to finish mixing the impression material.
- Larger fitting trays can be used.
- The impression material is injected through a tube on the front of the moulding tray when placed on the eye.
- Care should be taken to ensure that the cornea is not distorted by the injection process.
- The tray is gently lifted at its sides to ensure complete coverage of the globe.

Insertion method

- The moulding tray is filled with material before being placed on the eye with the head in a horizontal position.

- The patient's head remains horizontal until the material has set.

14.3.3 Producing the lens or shell

The impression is cast in dental stone to give a permanent positive cast of the eye.

Setting and making procedure

- A PMMA sheet is heat moulded over the cast, trimmed to size and edged.
- The optic zone clearance is worked using diamond-coated lapping tools.
- The substance removed from the centre to give minimum clearance is normally 0.15 mm, whereas 0.22 mm is taken from the limbal area.
- The optic zone is polished with wax tools or cloth-covered spherical brass tools.

Laboratory method

The cast is sent to a laboratory with the following specifications:

- BOZR. Either from a FLOM lens or 0.20 mm flatter than flattest 'K' [6]. Some laboratories can cope without specific directions and cut according to the cast.
- Back scleral size. Usually marked on the cast so that the optimum size is cut.
- BVP. From trial lens over-refraction.
- The transition is nearly always blended.
- Specifying centre thickness is unnecessary since it is determined from the other measurements. If altered, other parameters such as front optic radius are also changed.

14.3.4 Back vertex power

Over-refraction is carried out with a lens of known BOZR and BVP, preferably fitted slightly flat. A FLOM lens can be used if available. The front optic radius to give the required power is calculated and cut with a lathe.

14.3.5 Ventilation

Most patients can only wear a lens for a few hours before corneal hypoxia causes oedema. Ventilation allows fresh oxygenated tears to reach the cornea and is effected by:

- Fenestration, about 1 mm in diameter.
- Cutting a slot, usually 2 mm wide and one-quarter of the diameter of the limbus in length. It can be thinner if there is too much lid sensation.
- A channel of clearance connecting the optic zone to the lens.

In therapeutic fitting, however, scleral lenses are sometimes left sealed (i.e. not ventilated). This helps fluid retention where there is a tears deficiency and aids corneal coverage.

14.3.6 Scleral lenses with modern hard lens materials

Scleral lenses with modern hard lens materials are at an early stage, but experimental results suggest that there is a distinct improvement in corneal physiology compared with PMMA. Preformed sclerals can be lathed from large diameter buttons, and lenses made by the impression method can be duplicated using an individualized cast moulding system [7].

14.4 Scleral lens specification

The British Standards relating to sclerals are BS 5562:1978 and BS 3521:1988 Part 3 based on ISO 8320-1986.

For spherical preformed lenses:

BOZR = Back optic zone radius
BOZD = Back optic zone diameter
BPR = Back peripheral radius of optic, if present
POD = Primary optic diameter, where applicable
BSR = Back scleral radius
BSS = Back scleral size where specified is preceded by the letter B; otherwise TD is assumed
TD   = Total diameter
L   = Orientation of long axis in standard notation
D   = Displacement of optic and direction

Example (mm):

R /BOZR:BOZD/ BSR:BSS / L /D   /transition
R / 8.40:11.00 /13.00:B23.50/ L10 /D 1.00 in / sharp transitions

Some fitting sets still use the 1962 British Standards which gives a different specification:

Example (mm): 14.25/8.75/13.75/B23.50 D1 in.

Radius of back scleral surface   = 14.25
Radius of back optic zone   = 8.75
Primary optic diameter   = 13.75
Back scleral size or total diameter = B23.50
Displacement   = D1 in

References

1. Feinbloom, W. (1936) A plastic contact lens. *Transactions of the 15th Congress of the American Academy of Optometry*, **10**, 44
2. Cowan, J.M. (1948) The wide angle contact lens. *Optician*, **115**, 359
3. Bier, N. and Cole, P.J. (1948) The transcurve contact lens fitting shell. *Optician*, **115**, 605–610
4. Woodward, E.G. (1989) Preformed scleral lens fitting techniques. In *Contact Lenses*, A.J. Phillips and J. Stone (eds), Butterworths, London, pp. 625–644
5. Bier, N. (1948) The practice of ventilated contact lenses. *Optician*, **116**, 497–501
6. Pullum, K.W. (1989) Eye impressions, production and fitting of scleral lenses and patient management. In *Contact Lenses*, A.J. Phillips and J. Stone (eds), Butterworths, London, pp. 645–702
7. Pullum, K.W., Parker, J.H. and Hobley, A.J. (1989) Development of gas permeable scleral lenses produced from impressions of the eye; Josef Dallos Award Lecture 1989. *Transactions of the British Contact Lens Association Annual Clinical Conference*, **6**, 77–81.

Chapter 15

Soft lens design and fitting

The most appropriate design has to be selected from the very wide range of lens forms now available. Several factors must be taken into account:

- Size (corneal or semi-scleral).
- Water content (low, medium or high).
- Thickness (standard or thin) (*see* Section 17.4).
- Geometric and optic design (spherical or aspheric).
- Manufacturing method (lathed or moulded).
- Lens flexibility (*see* Section 17.2).
- Lens power (*see* Section 17.1).

All of these factors have some influence on vision, comfort and fitting characteristics, but the predominant factor which determines the method of fitting is usually the total diameter. The two main fitting philosophies into which soft lenses may be divided are therefore *corneal* and *semi-scleral*, although there is some degree of overlap with certain of the single diameter lenses.

15.1 Corneal diameter lenses

The majority of corneal diameter lenses are still manufactured from low to medium water materials to give reproducible lenses of good durability. The thinner varieties, in particular, cause minimum interference with corneal metabolism and give excellent cosmetic appearance.

Indications

- Most straightforward cases.
- Small corneas.

- Patients with small palpebral apertures and difficulty in handling.

Contraindications

- Very large corneas.
- Shallow corneoscleral junction allowing decentration.
- Tight lids causing lens decentration.
- Sensitive lid margin.
- Sensitive limbus.

FITTING

Radius

- Radius selection is based on keratometry.
- Most radii are between 7.90 mm and 8.90 mm.
- Less flexible low water content materials may require radii 0.70 mm or more flatter than 'K'.
- The radius for standard HEMA lenses is usually between 0.30 mm and 0.60 mm flatter than 'K'.
- High water content lenses are fitted closer to alignment.
- Fitting steps are usually between 0.20 mm and 0.40 mm.
- Most corneal lenses have a single curve back surface.

Total diameter

- Lenses should be just slightly larger than the horizontal visible iris diameter (HVID). They should extend beyond the limbus by up to 0.50–0.75 mm to avoid irritation.
- Most corneal lenses vary in size from 12.50–13.50 mm, with the possible range from 12.00–14.00 mm.
- High water content lenses are fitted approximately 0.50 mm larger than HEMA.
- High plus and high minus lenses are fitted approximately 0.50 mm larger than low powers in order to achieve stability on the cornea.
- Fitting steps are usually 0.50 mm.

Power

After allowing for vertex distance considerations, the lens power is usually within 0.25 D of the spectacle *Rx*. Thicker designs require about 0.25 D less minus than thin lenses.

Fitting appearance

Fitting characteristics are mainly as described in Chapter 16, but it is essential for a correctly fitting lens to give complete corneal coverage with proper centration to avoid the risk of epithelial dehydration and arcuate staining of any exposed area. The slit lamp should be used for careful observation of centration and movement, since these can be significantly influenced by factors such as:

- Corneal topography.
- Limbal topography.
- Lid pressure.
- Size of palpebral aperture.
- Position of cornea within palpebral aperture.

Figure 15.1 shows the four common ways in which a lens may position on the cornea with the eye in the primary position:

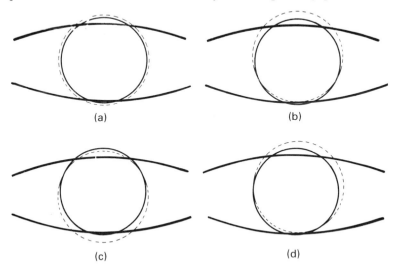

(a)   (b)

(c)   (d)

Figure 15.1 The four common positions (see text) taken up by soft lenses of corneal size, on an eye in the primary position: (a) correctly centred; (b) slightly high; (c) slightly low; (d) laterally decentred.

(a) An optimum fitting is shown. The lens is perfectly centred and there should be 0.50–1.00 mm of vertical movement on blinking.

(b) The lens is riding high, influenced perhaps by a tight upper lid. This may prove acceptable, provided that the decentration is no more than about 0.50 mm. An attempt should be made to improve the fitting by selecting a larger diameter.

(c) The lens is riding in a low position. It generally represents an unsatisfactory fitting which is either too small or too flat and the patient is likely to complain of unacceptable lid sensation. It can also occur with the downwards pressure of a relatively heavy upper lid. This creates a fitting which is too tight, although initially quite comfortable. There is the possibility, after several hours of wear, of arcuate staining at the superior limbus together with oedema from insufficient tears exchange.

(d) The lens is eccentrically located. This may also be due to a fitting which is too small or too flat, or because of lid pressure with a shallow corneoscleral junction. It represents an unsatisfactory fitting and a larger total diameter should be tried. However, if the decentration is limited to 0.50 mm, it may occasionally prove acceptable. An attempt should always be made to improve the fitting characteristics of a decentred lens by selecting a larger diameter. Where this fails, it may be necessary to consider a semi-scleral lens.

Clinical equivalents

The principle of clinical equivalents applies where two lenses of the same design and material, with different but related parameters, give similar fitting characteristics on the eye.

Rule of thumb

A change in diameter of 0.50 mm $\equiv$ a change in radius of 0.20 mm.

Examples: 7.90:12.50 $\equiv$ 8.10:13.00
8.30:13.00 $\equiv$ 8.50:13.50

To improve a loose fitting

● Select a larger total diameter.

• Select a steeper radius.

• Use a more rigid or lower water content material.

• Use a different lens thickness.

To improve a tight fitting

• Select a flatter radius.

• Select a smaller total diameter.

• Use a less rigid or higher water content material.

• Use a different lens thickness.

15.1.1 Examples of corneal diameter lenses

HYDRON MINI (ALLERGAN)

A standard thickness, corneal diameter lens for daily wear; manufactured by lathing.

Material properties

Chemical nature   HEMA cross-linked polymer
Water content   38.6% at 20°C
Dk 8.0×10^{-11} at 20°C
                   10.0×10^{-11} at 35°C
Refractive index   1.513 (dry), 1.43 (wet)

Lens geometry

• Centre thickness is 0.12 mm at −3.00 D and 0.21 mm at +2.00 D.

• Back surface is a single curve.

• Front surface is lenticulated.

Parameters available

See Table 15.1.

Table 15.1 Parameters available for Hydron Mini lenses

Radius (mm)	7.90–8.90 in 0.20 steps	8.10–9.30 in 0.20 steps
Diameter (mm)	12.50	13.00
Power (D)	±10.00 in 0.25 steps	
	±10.50 to ±30.00 in 0.50 steps	

Fitting technique

- Total diameter should be at least 1.00 mm larger than the HVID.
- Lenses of 13.00 mm diameter are used in about 90% of cases.
- Initial radius is selected approximately 0.70 mm flatter than 'K'.

Typical lens specification

8.70:13.00   −3.00

LUNELLE ES 70 (ESSILOR)

A high water content, corneal diameter lens for daily or extended wear; manufactured by lathing.

Material properties

Chemical properties	Copolymer of PMMA and polyvinyl pyrrolidone
Water content	70%
Dk	35.0×10^{-11} at 25°C
Refractive index	1.38

Lens geometry

- Centre thickness is 0.12 mm at −3.00 D; average thickness is 0.15 mm.
- Back surface is a single curve.
- Front surface is lenticulated.

Parameters available

See Table 15.2.

Table 15.2 Parameters available for Lunelle ES 70

Radius (mm)	7.70–8.30 in 0.30 steps	8.00–9.20 in 0.30 steps
Diameter (mm)	13.00	14.00
Power (D)	plano to −12.00	±20.00

Fitting technique

- The 14.00 mm diameter is selected for corneas larger than 11.25 mm; the 13.00 mm diameter for corneas 11.25 mm or smaller.
- The radius is selected to be at least 0.60 mm flatter than 'K' for 14.00 mm lenses and 0.30 mm flatter than 'K' for 13.00 mm lenses.
- Lens movement should be 1.00–1.50 mm.
- The relative stiffness of the material gives an advantage in correcting low to medium degrees of astigmatism (0.75–1.25 D).
- A low rate of lens dehydration is claimed to assist or avoid dry eye problems.

Typical lens specification

8.30:13.00   −3.00
8.90:14.00   −3.00

15.2 Semi-scleral lenses

The majority of lathed semi-sclerals are significantly larger and thicker than corneal soft lenses, giving better stability of both vision and fitting. In order to provide good physiological response, they are now mostly manufactured from medium to high water content materials with high Dk values.

Indications

- Most straightforward cases.
- Large corneas.
- Large palpebral apertures.
- Sensitive lid margin.
- Sensitive limbus.
- Hyperopes and high powers, if high water content.
- Moderate degrees of astigmatism (0.75–1.25 D).

Contraindications

- Very small corneas.

- Small palpebral apertures, if handling difficult.
- Corneas prone to oedema, if low water content.
- Where cosmetic appearance is important.

FITTING

Radius

- Radius selection is based on keratometry.
- Most radii are between 8.30 mm and 9.00 mm.
- High water content lenses are fitted between 0.30 mm and 1.00 mm flatter than 'K'.
- HEMA lenses are fitted flatter, between 0.70 mm and 1.30 mm flatter than 'K'.
- Fitting steps are usually 0.30 mm or 0.40 mm.
- Most semi-scleral lenses are of bicurve construction, with a relatively flat but narrow peripheral curve.

Total diameter

- Lenses are fitted significantly larger than the visible iris diameter, to give deliberate apical touch with further support beyond the limbus where they overlap onto the sclera. This type of three-point touch is shown in Figure 15.2.
- The total diameter is selected to be 2.00–3.00 mm larger than the horizontal visible iris diameter. However, many semi-scleral lenses are manufactured in only one size.
- The majority of semi-scleral lenses are fitted with total diameters of 14.30–14.80 mm; the possible range is from 13.50–16.00 mm.
- High water content and HEMA lenses are fitted with very similar diameters.
- Fitting steps are usually 0.50 mm.

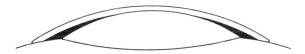

Figure 15.2 Semi-scleral lens giving three-point touch.

Power

Because of mainly flexure effects, the power of a correctly fitting lens often shows approximately 0.25–0.50 D less minus than the spectacle *Rx*, after allowing for any vertex distance considerations. With more rigid low water content lenses this can be as high as 0.75 D.

Fitting appearance

Fitting characteristics are mainly as described in Chapter 16 and Table 16.1. It is essential that a correctly fitting lens should be sufficiently large to span the limbus and not interfere with the blood vessels in this region.

Figure 15.3(a–c) shows diagrammatically the limits of acceptable movement and position for semi-scleral lenses with the eye in the primary position and in lateral and upward gaze. Figure 15.4(a–c) indicates the lack of movement with a tight lens, whereas Figure 15.5(a–c) shows the excessive mobility of a loose fitting.

Clinical equivalents and altering the fitting

The principle of clinical equivalents also applies so that two lenses of different but related specification behave in the same way on the eye.

Rule of thumb

A change in radius of 0.30 mm ≡ a change of diameter of 0.50 mm.

Examples: 8.10:13.50 ≡ 8.40:14.00
            8.70:14.50 ≡ 9.00:15.00

Clinical equivalents have approximately the same ratio of sagittal depth to total diameter. They do not have the same sagittal depth.

To improve a loose fitting

● Select a steeper radius.
● Select a larger total diameter.

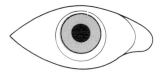

(a)

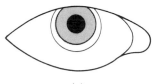

(b)

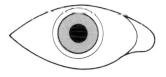

(c)

Figure 15.3 Appearance of a correctly fitting semi-scleral lens: (a) primary position; (b) lateral gaze; (c) upward gaze

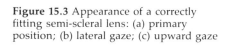

(a)

(b)

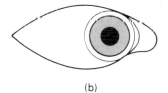

(c)

Figure 15.4 Appearance of a tightly fitting semi-scleral lens: (a) primary position; (b) lateral gaze; (c) upward gaze

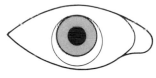

(a)

(b)

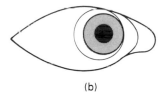

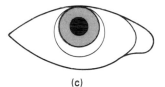

(c)

Figure 15.5 Appearance of a loose fitting semi-scleral lens: (a) primary position; (b) lateral gaze; (c) upward gaze

- Use a more rigid or lower water content material.
- Use a different lens thickness.

A lens of specification 8.70:14.00 may be progressively tightened with the following steps: 8.70:14.50; 8.40:14.00; 8.40:14.50.

To improve a tight fitting

- Select a flatter radius.
- Select a smaller total diameter.
- Use a less rigid or higher water content material.
- Use a different lens thickness.

A lens of specification 8.70:14.50 may be progressively loosened with the following steps: 8.70:14.00; 9.00:14.50; 9.00:14.00.

15.2.1 Examples of semi-scleral lenses

HYDROCURVE II 55 (PILKINGTON BARNES-HIND)

A medium water content, semi-scleral lens for daily or extended wear; manufactured by a combination of lathing and moulding.

Material properties

Chemical nature   Copolymer of HEMA, N-(1,1-dimethyl-3-oxo-
                   butylacrylamide) and methacrylic acid
Water content   55%
Dk 14.2×10^{-11} at 21°C
                   16.0×10^{-11} at 35°C
Refractive index   1.41

Lens geometry

- Centre thickness is 0.05 mm for a lens of power −3.00 D.
- Back surface is a moulded single curve.
- Front surface is lathed.

Parameters available

There are only two fittings available (Table 15.3).

Table 15.3 Parameters available for Hydrocurve II 55 lenses

Fittings (mm)	8.50:14.00, 8.80:14.50
Power (D)	+20.00 to −12.00

Fitting set

Lenses are provided in a range of powers for the two available fittings. The preferred method of fitting is from a lens stock.

Fitting technique

- The flatter fitting, 8.80:14.50, is used in the great majority of cases so that it is almost a 'one-fit' lens.
- The total diameter should be 1.50–2.00 mm larger than the HVID.
- If the lens is too flat, there is a tendency for the edge to buckle and give excessive lid sensation.

Typical specification

8.80:14.50   −3.00

PERMAFLEX (PILKINGTON BARNES-HIND)

A high water content, semi-scleral lens for daily or extended wear; manufactured by cast-moulding.

Material properties

Chemical nature   A cross-linked polymer of methyl methacrylate, vinyl pyrrolidone and other methacrylates
Water content   73.5%
Dk 34.0×10^{-11} at 25°C
   43.0×10^{-11} at 36°C
Refractive index   1.385

Lens geometry

- Centre thickness varies from 0.08 mm to 0.22 mm for minus powers; 0.14 mm for a −3.00 D lens.

- The back surface is a bicurve construction.
- 8.70 mm radii are spherical; 8.90 mm radii are aspheric.
- The front surface is lenticulated where necessary to give a minimum FOZD of 7.50 mm.

Parameters available

See Table 15.4.

Table 15.4 Parameters available for Permaflex

Radius (mm)	8.70		8.90
Diameter (mm)		14.40	
Power (D)	−10.00 to +8.00		plano to −10.00

Fitting technique

- The total diameter is constant at 14.40 mm.
- The spherical 8.70 mm radius fits a very high percentage of corneas so that it is almost a 'one-fit' lens.
- The 8.90 mm lenses are selected only for very flat or very small corneas.
- The 8.90 mm lenses fit significantly looser than would be expected because the back surface is aspheric and only *equivalent* to the designated radius.
- Because of the high water content, sufficient time must be allowed for lenses to settle, or an apparently correctly fitting may subsequently become tight.

Typical specification

8.70:14.40   −3.00

General advice

- Select the flatter of two possible fittings where there is a choice because:
  - (a) It is easier to see the movement of a lens which is too loose rather than the relative lack of movement of a steep fitting.
  - (b) A sharper end-point is obtained with over-refraction.

(c) Soft lenses become steeper and therefore tighter after initial settling.

- Steep corneas require lens selection to be relatively much flatter than flat corneas where the optimum result is likely to be much closer to 'K'. This applies to both corneal and semi-scleral lenses. Thus a radius of 8.10 mm may be necessary for a 13.00 mm lens on a 7.40 mm cornea, whereas an 8.40 mm cornea might well require a radius of 8.70 mm or perhaps 8.50 mm.

- It is better to achieve a more stable fitting by increasing the size. A steeper radius is likely to give worse acuity.

- It is essential to ensure adequate lens movement to allow proper exchange of tears and the removal of debris.

- It is also important to avoid fitting too tightly because of the risk of oedema. This can occur even with thin or high water content lenses.

Chapter 16

Soft lens fitting characteristics

Every make of lens has, to some extent, its own fitting characteristics. Most of the more general points, however, are summarized below, although the rather greater differences between corneal and semi-scleral lenses have been covered in Chapter 15.

16.1 Characteristics of a correct fitting

The general principles for a good fitting are complete corneal coverage, correct lens movement, good vision and comfort.

- 1 mm of vertical movement on blinking in primary position.
- Lag of up to 1.5 mm on upwards gaze or lateral eye movements.
- Good centration.
- Comfortable in all directions of gaze.
- Complete corneal coverage.
- Good visual acuity.
- Retinoscopy reflex crisp and sharp before and after blinking.
- Vision remains stable on blinking.
- Refraction gives a precise end-point.
- Refraction correlates with spectacle BVP.
- Keratometer mires stable and undistorted.
- No irritation of limbal vessels.
- No compression of bulbar conjunctiva.

16.2 Characteristics of a tight fitting

The obvious feature of a tight lens is insufficient movement. Initial comfort is therefore good and sometimes better than a correct fitting. Centration is also usually good, although a corneal diameter lens may sometimes assume a decentred position. This is easily differentiated from a decentred flat fitting because of the lack of movement. A steep lens vaults the corneal apex, but is momentarily pressed onto the eye by blinking to give a transient improvement in vision.

- Little or no movement on blinking (less than 0.5 mm).
- Little or no movement on upwards or lateral gaze (less than 0.5 mm).
- Good centration.
- Good initial comfort.
- Subsequent symptoms of discomfort such as heat or stinging.
- Poor visual acuity.
- Retinoscopy reflex shows irregular distortion.
- Unstable vision with temporary improvement on blinking.
- Refraction difficult with poor end-point.
- More negative power required than anticipated because of flexure or possible liquid lens.
- Keratometer mires give irregular distortion.
- Irritation of limbal or conjunctival vessels.
- Compression ring in bulbar conjunctiva (scleral indentation), often seen after the lens is removed.

16.3 Characteristics of a loose fitting

The obvious feature of a loose lens is excessive movement. On looking upwards it may catch against the top lid and cause noticeable discomfort. In the primary position, lower lid sensation is experienced if the lens sags, and the discomfort is accentuated if the fitting is so flat that the periphery buckles to give edge stand-off (Figure 16.1).

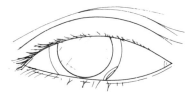

Figure 16.1 Very loose fitting showing buckling of lens edge

- Excessive movement on blinking (over 2 mm).
- Excessive lag on lateral or upwards eye movements (over 3 mm).
- Poor centration.
- Poor comfort because of lid sensation.
- Visual acuity variable.
- Retinoscopy reflex clear centrally with peripheral distortion.
- Variable vision.
- Refraction variable because of lens movement.
- Keratometer mires vary with lens movement, giving peripheral distortion.
- Buckling of lens edge.

16.4 Summary of soft lens fitting characteristics

The general fitting characteristics for soft lenses are summarized in Table 16.1.

Table 16.1 Fitting characteristics of soft lenses

Characteristic	Good fit	Steep fit	Flat fit
Comfort	Good	Good, initially	Poor
Centration	Good, with complete corneal coverage	Usually good, may be decentred, no recovery on blinking	Poor
Movement on blinking	Up to 1.0 mm	Less than 0.5 mm	Excessive, over 2.0 mm
Movement on upwards gaze	Up to 1.5 mm	Little or none	Excessive, over 3.0 mm
Movement on lateral gaze	Up to 1.5 mm	Little or none	Excessive, over 3.0 mm
Vision	Good	Poor and variable, momentary improvement on blinking	Variable, may improve on staring after blinking
Over-refraction	Precise end-point, power correlates with BVP of spectacle Rx	Poorly defined end-point, positive liquid lens	Variable, negative liquid lens

Table 16.1 *continued*

Characteristic	Good fit	Steep fit	Flat fit
Retinoscopy reflex	Clear reflex, before and after blinking	Poor and distorted, central shadow, momentarily improved on blinking	Variable, may be clear centrally with peripheral distortion
Slit lamp after settling	No limbal injection or scleral indentation	Conjunctival or limbal injection, scleral indentation	Localized limbal injection, possible edge stand-off
Keratometer mires	Sharp, stable before and after blinking	Irregular, momentary improvement on blinking	Variable and eccentric, changing on blinking
Placido disc	Regular image	Irregular image anywhere but at the edge of the lens	Irregular image, more often peripheral only but occasionally central as well

Chapter 17

Other soft lens fitting considerations

17.1 Lens power

Power is an important consideration in deciding which type of lens to fit.

Low minus (< −2.00 D)

- Thin lenses should be avoided because of handling difficulties.
- A thicker, medium or high water content lens should be selected.

High minus (> −7.00 D) and medium to high plus (> +3.00 D)

- Low water content lenses should be avoided because of the greater thickness and physiological problems.
- Semi-scleral lenses usually give better stability of fitting.

Medium minus (−2.00 D to −7.00 D) and low plus (< +3.00)

- Thin or high water content lenses are the probable choice, except where problems arise with fitting characteristics, dehydration or vision.

17.2 Lens flexibility

An important influence on the fitting characteristics of all lenses is the flexibility of the material. This explains why two lenses of apparently the same specification but different material can behave in entirely different ways on the cornea [1]. Permalens, for example, which is very flexible, often requires to be fitted steeper than 'K' compared with other more rigid materials where the more usual flatter than 'K' approach is correct. Similarly, thin spun-cast lenses and moulded lenses with overall a thin cross-section and inherently greater flexibility than their lathed counterparts lend themselves better to a 'one-fit' fitting philosophy which relies on draping the cornea.

Practical advice

- Because of flexibility and manufacturing considerations, the lenses from one laboratory cannot necessarily be duplicated by another, merely by ordering the same nominal specification.
- Fitting must be carried out with trial lenses of the type to be ordered.

17.3 Additional visual considerations

Flexure and liquid lens power

Flexure occurs when a soft lens fitted flatter or steeper than 'K' bends to follow the corneal curvature. The refractive effect with either plus or minus lenses is to add negative power [2,3].

A liquid lens occurs if the posterior surface of the soft lens fails to conform to the front surface of the cornea [4]. This is more likely to be present with semi-scleral designs, whereas there is virtually no liquid lens with ultra-thin lenses which completely drape the cornea.

Practical advice

- Any discrepancy between contact lens and spectacle *Rx* (allowing for vertex distance) is caused mainly by flexure but possibly by liquid lens power.
- This is unlikely to be greater than 0.50 D with a satisfactory fitting.
- Thin corneal lenses require more minus power than thick semi-scleral lenses.

Astigmatism

The usual limit for acceptable acuity with a thin spherical lens is about 1.00 DC, but it can be as little as 0.50 DC for critical observers. Very occasionally, acceptable vision is obtained with cylinders as high as 4.00 D and with an amblyopic eye there may be no advantage in the additional complexity and cost of a toric lens.

Soft lenses are generally fitted flatter than 'K' so that less minus is required compared with the best vision sphere used with hard lenses. Example:

Spectacle Rx −3.50/−1.00 × 180
Likely BVP of spherical soft lens −3.50 D.

Environmental factors

The power of a soft lens depends on its basic dimension of radius, diameter, thickness and refractive index which can all vary with environmental factors. These include ocular effects such as temperature, pH, tonicity and volume of tears. Some of these are in turn influenced by external factors such as ambient temperature, humidity, or the degree of lens hydration when placed on the eye. Generally, HEMA undergoes smaller changes than high water content materials and gives less variation in vision.

17.4 Thin lenses

Lenses with a centre thickness less than 0.10 mm may be regarded as 'thin' (*see* Section 5.3.2). Lenses in the range 0.05–0.07 mm are 'ultra-thin' and those less than 0.05 mm are 'hyperthin'.

The fitting characteristics of thin and standard lenses differ even if having otherwise identical specification. Lens thickness may therefore be regarded as an additional fitting variable.

In practical terms, thin lenses generally

● Possess greater flexibility.

● Prove easier to fit because there are fewer fitting steps.

● Drape the cornea more completely and give less mobility.

● Give less lid sensation and are more comfortable.

● Have better transmissibility (Dk/t).

- Possess different fitting characteristics and sometimes permit better centration.
- Give less satisfactory acuity on toric corneas.
- Dehydrate to a greater extent on the eye after settling.

HYDROFLEX SD (WOHLK)

A thin HEMA, corneal diameter lens for daily wear (the thin version of the standard thickness Hydroflex/m); manufactured by lathing.

Material properties

Chemical nature   HEMA
Water content   38.6%
Dk 7.3×10^{-11} at 21°C
                  8.1×10^{-11} at 35°C
Refractive index 1.448 at 23°C

Lens geometry

- All minus lenses have a centre thickness of 0.08 mm and an edge thickness of 0.05 mm.
- The back surface is a single curve.
- The front surface is lenticulated to give a constant FOZD of 7.80 mm for both plus and minus lenses.

Parameters available

See Table 17.1

Table 17.1 Parameters available for Hydroflex SD lenses

	Low powers	Aphakic powers
Radius (mm)	7.60–8.80 in 0.40 steps	8.40–9.20 in 0.40 steps
Diameter (mm)	13.00, 13.50	14.50
Power (D)	±10.00 in 0.25 steps	+14.00 to +20.00 in 0.25 steps

Fitting technique

- 13.50 mm is the most commonly used diameter.

- 13.00 mm lenses are used for small corneas or where the larger diameter causes lower lid sensation.
- Radius is selected to be 0.30–0.50 mm flatter than 'K'.
- The large fitting intervals of 0.40 mm work well because of the lens flexibility.
- Lens movement should be 0.50–1.00 mm.

Typical specification

Hydroflex SD: 8.40:13.50   −3.00

HYDRON ZERO 6 AND Z PLUS (ALLERGAN-HYDRON)

Thin HEMA, semi-scleral lenses for daily wear; manufactured by lathing.

Material properties

HEMA 38.6% (*see* Section 15.1).

Lens geometry

- Centre thickness is 0.06 mm for all minus lenses of power −3.00 D or greater.
- The mid-periphery is deliberately thickened to make handling easier.
- Z Plus lenses have an *average* thickness of 0.10 mm.
- The back surface is a bicurve with a constant BOZD of 13.28 mm and peripheral curve width of 0.36 mm (13.28 mm + 0.36 mm + 0.36 mm = 14.00 mm).
- The front surface is lenticulated with BOZDs of 6.70 mm at −10.00 D and 8.3 mm at +10.00 D.

Parameters available

See Table 17.2.

Table 17.2 Parameters available for Hydron Zero 6 and Z Plus lenses

Radius (mm)	8.40, 8.70, 9.00 (8.10, 9.30 also made)
Diameter (mm)	14.00
Power (D)	±20.00

Fitting technique

- Approximately 70% of minus lenses are fitted with the 8.70 mm radius.
- The most common radius for Z Plus lenses is 9.00 mm.
- There is no very firm relationship between 'K' and radius because of greater lens flexibility.
- 14.00 mm is the only available diameter. Lenses may prove unsuitable if the cornea is either very large or very small.

Typical specification

Zero 6: 8.70:14.00   −3.00
Z Plus: 9.00:14.00   +3.00

17.5 Aspheric lenses

Back surface aspherics

A minority of soft lenses have an aspheric back surface designed to match the aspheric nature of the cornea. A correctly fitting lens behaves in the main as described in Section 16.1 but compared with spherical lenses:

- Aspherics do not have a true radius but are designated in some other way such as by 'fitting value' or posterior apical radius (PAR).
- Changing the total diameter does not necessarily alter the fitting characteristics.
- Lens mobility of between 0.50 mm and 2.00 mm can be acceptable.
- With some corneal geometries proper centration cannot be achieved and a spherical lens is required, although the reverse is also true.

WEICON CE (60%) (CIBA VISION)

A back surface aspheric, corneal diameter lens for daily or extended wear; manufactured by CNC lathes.

Material properties

Chemical nature   Methyl methacrylate/vinyl pyrrolidone (MMA/VP) copolymer

Water content   60%
Dk 28×10^{-11} at 35°C
Refractive index   1.4037

Lens geometry

- Centre thickness of a $-3.00\,D$ lens is $0.09\,mm$.
- All lenses have an elliptical back surface with a 'flat' (FL) or 'steep' (ST) 'fitting value' instead of a radius.
- Radius and eccentricity are varied to give a consistent performance throughout the power range.
- Lenses feature a 'tangential bevel' to give a continuous transition between back surface and ski-shaped edge.

Parameters available

See Table 17.3.

Table 17.3 Parameters available for Weicon 38E lenses

Fitting value (eccentricity)	Flat (FL) or steep (ST)
Diameter (mm)	13.00, 13.80, 14.60
Power (D)	±25.00

Fitting technique

- The $13.80\,mm$ diameter is most commonly used.
- The FL fitting value is generally selected.
- The ST fitting value is tried only if the FL is excessively mobile after complete settling.

Typical specification

Weicon CE 60%: FL 13.80 -3.00

Front surface aspherics

A front surface aspheric (e.g. Nissel SV38) can give improved acuity in cases of low to medium astigmatism ($0.75-1.50\,D$) by the correction of optical aberrations.

17.6 Spun-cast lenses

SOFLENS (BAUSCH AND LOMB)

Corneal and semi-scleral lenses for daily wear; manufactured by spin-casting in open moulds.

Material properties

Chemical nature	HEMA cross-linked polymer
Water content	38.6%
Dk	8.0×10^{-11} at 20°C
Refractive index	1.43

Lens geometry

- The front surface gives the 'series' or 'base curve', determined by the constant curvature of the mould during manufacture. This is the opposite of conventional lathed lenses (typical series are shown in Figure 17.1).
- The back surface is aspheric and governs the power (Figure 17.2).
- Most of the minus series have constant sag and centre thickness, irrespective of power (*see* Table 17.4).
- The higher the minus power, the tighter the fitting.
- Series are designated according to thickness and size. The suffix '4' denotes a 14.50 mm diameter; the suffix '3' a 13.50 mm diameter; and where there is no numerical suffix (e.g. U and the original F series), a 12.50 mm diameter.

ADVANTAGES OF SPIN-CASTING

- Better surface quality and edge shape.
- Mass production ensures better reproducibility and consistency of manufacture.

Disadvantages of spin-casting

- Limitations on the variety of back surface forms which may be conveniently obtained.
- The full power range is not obtainable for each series.

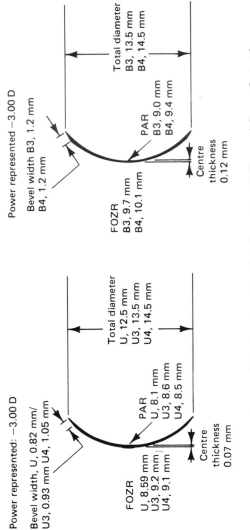

Figure 17.1 Two typical series of the Bausch and Lomb Soflens (from Phillips and Stone, *Contact Lenses*, 3rd edn, Butterworth-Heinemann, by permission)

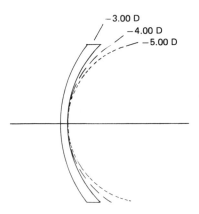

-3.00 D
-4.00 D
-5.00 D

Figure 17.2 Bausch and Lomb Soflens. The front surface radius is constant. Variation in power is achieved by altering the posterior apical radius: the steeper it is, the higher the negative power

Parmeters available

See Table 17.4.

Table 17.4 Parameters available for Bausch and Lomb Soflens lenses

Lens series	Power range (D)	Diameter (mm)	Centre thickness (mm)	Sag (mm)
Sofspin	−0.25 to −12.00	14.00	0.05–0.09	
U	−0.25 to −9.00	12.50	0.07	2.89
U3	−9.00 to +6.00	13.50	0.07–0.18	3.09
U4	−9.00 to +6.00	14.50	0.07–0.18	4.05
L3	−0.25 to −3.00	13.50	0.06	3.09
L4	−0.25 to −3.00	14.50	0.06	3.65
B3	−20.00 to +6.00	13.50	0.12–0.30	3.10 (3.20*)
B4	−9.00 to +6.00	14.50	0.12–0.30	3.59
O3	−1.00 to 9.00	13.50	0.035	3.18 (3.12†)
O4	−1.00 to −9.00	14.50	0.035	4.10 (3.68‡)
F	−0.25 to −9.50	12.50	0.18	2.84
M3	+3.00 to +14.00	13.50	0.23–0.44	3.41–3.61
M4	+3.00 to +14.00	14.50	0.23–0.44	3.66–3.86
N (non-lenticulated)	+0.25 to +6.00	12.50	0.18–0.36	3.86–4.02
N	+6.50 to +18.50	13.50	0.40–0.75	
H3	+10.00 to +20.00	13.50	0.48–0.61	3.40–3.47
H4	+10.00 to +20.00	14.50	0.48–0.61	3.69–3.80
HO3	−8.00 to −20.00	13.50	0.035	3.61
HO4	−8.00 to −20.00	14.50	0.035	3.67
Optima 38	−0.25 to −6.00	14.00	0.06	3.60/3.82

Except:
*−12.50 to −20.00; †−1.00 to −1.25; ‡−1.00 to −1.75.

Fitting technique

- The constant sag and the greater flexibility of spun lenses effectively give a 'one-fit' approach for each particular series.
- Fitting characteristics depend upon total diameter, thickness and power.
- Diameter is chosen on the basis of corneal size. 13.50 mm lenses (3 series) are used where HVID is less than 11.75 mm, and 14.50 mm (4 series) where it is greater.
- Series and thickness are selected according to physiological and handling considerations.
- Power is based on spectacle *Rx* and vertex distance.
- If adequate centration cannot be achieved with the initial diameter, the next larger lens with the same letter series should be tried (e.g. if U3 is too small, change to U4).
- It is particularly important to achieve complete corneal coverage or there is a likelihood of arcuate staining at the limbus from corneal drying and edge abrasion.
- Lens decentration is likely to give poor vision because of the aspheric optics.
- Decentration can occur with either a loose or a tight fitting, but in the latter case there is no recovery movement on blinking.
- Movement on blinking is only about 0.50 mm (i.e. less than most other lenses).
- Other fitting characteristics are mainly as described in Chapter 16.
- Plus lenses are selected according to similar principles, although centre thickness varies according to power.
- The plus power range is divided into three overlapping groups, each with a different sag.

USING THE DIFFERENT SERIES

U3 and U4 ($t_c = 0.07$ mm)

The most commonly used series.

Typical specification

Soflens: -3.00 U4

O series (t_c = 0.035 mm)

Where greater transmissibility is required for extended wear. However, they are extremely difficult to handle and have a tendency to dehydrate more readily on the eye (*see* Sections 5.3.3 and 20.4.2).

B series (t_c = 0.12 mm)

For easier handling and to provide an extension to the power range.

L series (t_c = 0.06 mm)

For low minus powers up to −3.00 D. Designed to be ultra-thin in the centre, with a relatively thicker peripheral geometry to permit easier handling than either O or U series of the same diameter.

HO series (t_c = 0.035 mm)

For high minus powers. The large FOZD, despite lenticulation, gives a relatively thick periphery, so these lenses are not always ideal for cases prone to vascularization.

F series (t_c = 0.18 mm)

For very small corneas where handling difficulties arise with the 12.50 mm U series.

Sofspin (t_c = 0.05–0.09 mm)

Where a variable centre thickness is required with a single diameter (14.00 mm) for ease of fitting.

Optima (t_c = 0.06 mm)

Where greater rigidity and ease of handling are required. The back surface is lathed and there are two possible sags. Sag I (3.60 mm) gives greater movement and is fitted with flatter corneas; Sag II (3.82 mm) gives better centration and is used with steeper corneas.

17.7 'One-fit' lenses

Most 'one-fit' lenses are semi-scleral in type. They can give a satisfactory result in a high percentage of cases because of their large diameter, thinness and flexibility.

- Because no fitting adjustment is possible, it is important to recognize early those cases for whom the fitting characteristics fail to meet the criteria given in Chapter 16.
- With thinner varieties, especially spun-cast lenses, limited lens mobility of only 0.50 mm may be acceptable.
- To assess the fitting reliably, trial lenses should be as near as possible to the correct power.
- Particular care is required with corneas which are unusually small, large, steep or flat.

HYDROFIT (CANTOR AND SILVER)

A single fitting, thin HEMA, semi-scleral lens for daily wear; manufactured by computer-controlled automatic lathes.

Material properties

HEMA 38%.

Lens geometry

- Centre thickness for minus lenses varies between 0.05 mm and 0.07 mm.
- Edge thickness is 0.15 mm.
- BOZR and total diameter are constant for all lenses.
- Back surface is a bicurve with a 10.75 mm peripheral radius.
- Front surface is lenticulated with a junction thickness of 0.20 mm.

Parameters available

See Table 17.5

Table 17.5 Parameters available for Hydrofit lenses

Radius (mm)	8.80
Diameter (mm)	14.50
Power (D)	±20.00

Fitting technique

- Fitting is assessed with lenses as near as possible to the correct power.

Typical specification

Hydrofit: 8.80:14.50   −3.00

17.8 Unusual lens performance

Fitting sometimes gives unexpected or unreliable results. If the lens is:

Too tight

- Stored in *hypotonic* solution, giving temporary osmotic adhesion.
- Causing initial irritation with excessive lacrimation and a hypotonic shift in the patient's tears.
- Ultra-thin with a temporarily distorted shape because it has adhered to the base, neck or lid of the storage vial.
- Disinfected by heat without sufficient time to cool and revert to its proper dimensions.

Too loose

- Stored in *hypertonic* solution.
- Inserted inside out.
- Damaged.

References

1. Gasson, A.P. (1989) Soft (hydrogel) lens fitting. In *Contact Lenses*, A.J. Phillips and J. Stone (eds), Butterworths, London, pp. 382–439
2. Bennett, A.G. (1976) Power changes in soft lenses due to bending. *Ophthalmic Optician*, **16**, 939–945
3. Sarver, M.D., Ashley, D. and Van Every, J. (1974) Supplemental power effect of Bausch and Lomb Softlens contact lenses. *International Contact Lens Clinic*, **1**, 100–109
4. Wichterle, O. (1967) Changes of refracting power of a soft lens caused by its flattening. In *Corneal and Scleral Contact Lenses*, Proceedings of the International Congress, L.J. Girard (ed.), paper 29, Mosby, St. Louis, pp. 247–256.

Chapter 18

Frequent (planned) replacements and disposable lenses

Considerably fewer clinical difficulties arise when lenses are replaced on a regular basis. Deposits are avoided and there are much reduced risks of discomfort, PC, infections and red eyes (*see* Chapter 27). It has always been difficult to define the life span of a soft lens because it depends on a variety of factors:

- Water content and material.
- Lens thickness.
- Method of disinfection and cleaning.
- Wearing time.
- Daily or extended wear.
- Tear chemistry.
- Handling ability.
- Environment.

A reasonable average before lenses need either replacement or thorough professional cleaning is about 12 months. Many practitioners and laboratories have therefore devised schemes which encourage patients by means of relatively reduced fees to replace lenses on a frequent and planned basis before they reach the troublesome stage.

The replacement interval depends upon the practitioner, patient and make of lens, but is typically set at 12, 6 or 3 months. The ultimate of frequent replacement is the 'disposable lens' which is discarded and replaced for a very modest fee on a much more frequent basis, usually weekly, fortnightly or monthly. Lenses were originally developed for extended wear, but they also have significant advantages even for purely daily wear.

18.1 Advantages and disadvantages of disposable lenses

ADVANTAGES

- Lenses rarely reach the stage where they build up deposits.
- Reduced risk of allergies and infections.
- Reduced incidence of papillary conjunctivitis (PC).
- Safer and better for most extended wear (*see* Chapter 20).
- Spare lenses are always available.
- Replacement cost is significantly less if lost or damaged.
- Less time and effort required with lens cleaning.
- Cost savings on solutions.
- Patients like the regular fresh feeling of new lenses.
- Easy to fit, since fitting parameters are very limited.
- Ideal for children requiring soft lenses.
- Easy to cope with power changes.

DISADVANTAGES

- Restricted range of fittings and powers.
- Inappropriate for complex lenses such as torics or bifocals.
- Increased cost on an annual basis.
- Inadequate control over patient compliance.
- In the event of a clinical problem, patients may merely replace lenses rather than seek professional advice.
- Not feasible to check every lens.
- Administrative complexities because of the volume of lenses.

18.2 Other uses of disposable lenses

The low unit cost of disposables means that they have other very useful clinical applications apart from normal daily and extended wear.

- Low cost temporary replacement in emergency.
- Maintaining soft lens wear when PC is causing rapid deposits.
- Short-term use in the hay fever season to avoid PC.

- Periodic use for patients working with VDUs intensively but intermittently.

- Where an approximate contact lens refraction is needed for a patient with an eye infection and the practitioner would not wish to contaminate a conventional trial lens.

- To give a lengthy tolerance trial for contact lenses in general (e.g. can the patient cope with handling and disinfection?).

- To give an extended assessment of contact lens vision (e.g. can monovision be tolerated?).

- To assess the patient's reaction, over several days, to the lens material in terms of dehydration and comfort prior to ordering in conventional lens form.

- As a means of assessing children who require soft lenses.

18.3 Fitting and aftercare

- Fitting principles follow those described in Chapters 15–17.

- Lenses are either 'one-fit' or very limited in parameters, so that it is important to recognize when a satisfactory fitting cannot be achieved.

- It is essential to avoid tight lenses if they are to be used for extended wear.

- Aftercare follows the normal principles described in Chapter 27, for both daily and extended wear.

- Intervals for routine aftercare visits are arranged to coincide with the dispensing of lens supplies.

Chapter 19

Soft lens specification and verification

19.1 British and International Standards

The British Standards document on soft lenses (3521:Part 3:1988 replacing BS 3521:1979), at the time of writing, covers only terminology. This derives from International Standard ISO 8320-1986 which also covers hard lenses.

19.2 Lens specification

A typical soft lens specification takes the following abbreviated form:

8.40:13.50   −3.00   HEMA   38% water content

where   8.40 = back optic zone radius (BOZR),
   13.50 = total diameter (TD),
   −3.00 = BVP.

The majority of lenses are made according to predetermined laboratory designs and it is neither necessary nor feasible to specify parameters such as thickness, lenticulation and peripheral curves (Chapters 15 and 17 include other examples).

19.3 Soft lens verification

Soft lenses require verification for the same reasons as hard (see Section 11.3) although checking is considerably more difficult because parameters vary with:

- Degree of hydration.
- Temperature.
- pH and tonicity of storage solution.
- Nature of the storage solution.

- Time taken if measurement is in air.
- Method of supporting lens.

19.3.1 Back optic zone radius

SPHEROMETERS

Many common methods of radius checking rely on the principle of spherometry, where the sagittal depth is measured for a given chord diameter. The majority of instruments employ a wet cell, but this is not essential.

Wet cell instruments (e.g. Optimec)

- The lens is rinsed and placed in a wet cell containing 0.9% saline solution.
- The lens is centred on a support device.
- A probe is advanced towards the concave surface until it just touches (established by viewing lens movement or electric contact) and the radius is read from the instrument scale.

Measurement in air (e.g. Wöhlk spherometer)

- The lens is rinsed in saline; surplus fluid is removed by shaking and rapid superficial drying.
- The lens is centred on a 10 mm support ring, concave side down.
- The central probe is observed from above through a magnifying lens until the first point of contact is made and the radius is read from instrument scale.

OTHER METHODS

Base curve comparator

A simple device consisting of a series of spheres of known radius on which the contact lens is placed and compared by straightforward observation in air.

A much more sophisticated wet cell instrument by Söhnges allows the profile of the lens to be matched with known radii on a projection screen.

Keratometer

This can be used in conjunction with a wet cell [1]. Measured radius, however, requires conversion to actual radius and observation is difficult because the light intensity is considerably reduced [2].

19.3.2 Total diameter

PROJECTION MAGNIFIERS

An optical system projects a magnified image of the lens onto a calibrated screen. Instruments may use a wet cell (e.g. Optimec, Söhnges) or support the lens in air on a microscope stage (e.g. Zeiss DL2).

COMPARISON

Comparators consisting of a series of annuli of known diameter can be used as a rapid in-air method.

19.3.3 Power

AIR MEASUREMENT

- Rinse the lens with saline.
- Shake off surplus fluid and dry carefully with a lint-free tissue.
- Place lens concave surface down on a reduced aperture focimeter stop.
- Read power directly from focimeter scale.

WET CELL MEASUREMENT

- Place lens in wet cell.
- Mount on focimeter.
- Read power from focimeter scale.
- Convert to approximate power in air by multiplying by four [3].

Practical advice

- Power is more easily and more accurately measured in air.
- Any error in wet cell measurement is magnified fourfold (an error of 0.25 D ≡ 1.00 D in air).
- Power in air is reasonably constant for about 2 min.
- Best results are obtained with a projection focimeter.

19.3.4 Thickness

PROJECTION MAGNIFIERS

The easiest method of measuring thickness is by means of a millimetre scale calibrated for the screen of a projection magnifier (e.g. Optimec, Söhnges).

DRYSDALE'S METHOD

A hard lens radiuscope can be used to determine lens thickness [4]:

- Place the lens, concave surface down, on a convex sphere (this should have a curvature steeper than the lens to be measured to ensure contact at the centre).
- Focus the target on the surface of the sphere with the lens in place.
- Set the scale to zero.
- Focus the target on the front surface of the lens.
- Read the distance travelled from the scale.
- Multiply by the refractive index of the material to give the actual centre thickness.

19.3.5 Edge form

Edge form and integrity are best observed with projection magnification, but a hand loupe or the slit lamp can also be used.

19.3.6 Surface quality

Surface quality is assessed with the slit lamp or by means of projection magnification. Observation with a wet cell is more difficult because the small difference in the refractive index of the solution largely disguises any surface flaws or cracks.

19.3.7 Water content and material

Water content can be estimated with a refractometer because of its inverse relationship with refractive index. An instrument developed for contact lens measurement is the Atago CL-1 refractometer [5].

- Rinse the hydrated lens with saline, shake off surplus moisture and blot with a lint-free tissue.
- Flatten lens against prism face, taking care not to cause damage.
- Use an external light source and read directly from the internal scale the water content at the junction between light and dark areas.

Assessing the lens material from the water content alone is far from certain, so identification may depend upon other clues such as style of engraving (see Section 24.1), handling tint or type of edge bevel.

19.3.8 Deposits

Projection magnifiers reveal discrete areas of deposit such as white spots. Films such as protein are more easily observed by looking into the wet cell without magnification. The best method of observing deposits, however, is by dark field illumination [6].

High magnification can be achieved with the slit lamp by using an oblique beam and selecting a dark background. In addition, some lens deposits fluoresce with ultraviolet light.

Practical advice

- The easiest methods for practitioner verification are:

BOZR	Wet cell or in-air spherometer
DIAMETER	Projection magnifier
POWER	Focimeter in air
THICKNESS	Projection magnifier
CONDITION	Projection magnifier

- The most useful instrument, which is ideally kept in the consulting room, is a projection magnifier. It is not only used for lens inspection, but also for demonstrating to the patient surface and edge flaws and deposits.
- Wet cells are a source of possible cross-infection and require regular cleaning and disinfection.
- Particular care is required when flattening high water content lenses against a glass surface (e.g. microscope stage or refractometer) because of the difficulty of removal and the risk of damage.

19.4 Tolerances

At the time of writing, British and International Standards have not published a document on soft lens tolerances. A fairly lenient American Standard, however, was produced in 1986 [7].

Table 19.1 gives tolerances that are recommended as reasonably consistent with the accuracy of current instruments for soft lens verification.

Table 19.1 Recommended tolerances for soft lenses

BOZR	± 0.15 mm
Total diameter	± 0.20 mm
Thickness	± 0.02 mm
BVP (plano to 6.00 D)	± 0.12 D
(>6.00 D)	± 0.25 D

References

1. Loran, D.F.C. (1989) The verification of hydrogel contact lenses. In *Contact Lenses*, A.J. Phillips and J. Stone (eds), Butterworths, London, pp. 463–504
2. Chaston, J. (1973) A method of measuring the radius of curvature of a soft contact lens. *Optician*, **165**, 8–12
3. Poster, M.G. (1971) Hydrated method of determining dioptric power of all hydrophilic lenses. *Journal of the American Optometric Association*, **43**, 287–299
4. Hartstein, J. (1973) *Questions and Answers on Contact Lens Practice*, 2nd edn, Mosby, St. Louis, pp. 155–157
5. Efron, N. and Brennan, N.A. (1987) The soft contact lens refractometer. *Optician*, **94**(5115), 29–41
6. Killpartrick, M.R. (1987) Soft lens contaminant detection by dark field illumination. *Optician*, **193**(5083), 34–37
7. American National Standard (1986) Prescription requirements for first quality soft contact lenses. In *American National Standard Requirements for Soft Contact Lenses 280.8 – 1986*, National Standards Institute for Ophthalmics, USA

Chapter 20

Extended wear

Soft lenses have been routinely fitted for extended wear since the early 1970s with the introduction of Permalens and Sauflon PW. Improvements have since occurred not only in lens design but also in the understanding of the physiological requirements of the cornea necessary to achieve extended wear with relative safety. More recently, high Dk hard lenses have also been introduced with some advantage.

20.1 Physiological requirements

20.1.1 Oxygen requirements of the cornea

Limiting any hypoxic effect on the cornea is essential for successful long-term wear of any contact lens. In practical terms for extended wear, the following physiological requirements must be met [1]:

First day of extended wear Dk/t for zero swelling $= 24 \times 10^{-9}$
Second day of extended wear Dk/t for zero swelling $= 34 \times 10^{-9}$
For overnight swelling of only 4%, Dk/t $= 87 \times 10^{-9}$

No soft lens is able to fulfil these criteria, since the theoretical limit, with current materials, is a Dk of approximately 40×10^{-11}.

Hard lens materials, however, are available with at least double the permeability of high water content soft lenses before taking into account any tears pump effect. Lenses with a Dk in the region of 100 (e.g. Fluorofocon) provide approximately 15% EOP.

The tears pump adds about 2% oxygen to give a total EOP of 17% for open eye conditions and 4% for closed eye. This is sufficient to avoid epithelial compromize in extended wear with most patients [2].

173

20.1.2 Effects of insufficient oxygen

Extended wear causes chronic cumulative hypoxia to a much greater extent than daily wear because of continuous eye closure during sleep, with sometimes inadequate time for corneal deswelling during the day. Between 10% and 15% oxygen is needed to avoid oedema and measurable corneal changes [3].

- Epithelial changes include decreased glycolysis [4], decreased mitosis [5], decreased cell adhesion [6] and reduced sensitivity [7].
- The stroma shows oedema which eventually leads to stromal thinning [4].
- Endothelial cells show distinct polymegathous changes similar to those seen in the 'corneal exhaustion syndrome' [4].

20.1.3 Tears exchange and osmolarity

There is a normal increase in corneal thickness overnight, mainly due to a change in tear osmolarity causing swelling. This rapidly disappears on eye opening. Soft lens materials may become tighter with these changes and lens adhesion may be found in the morning. Lenses usually start moving after a few blinks and this movement is very important to allow tears exchange to eliminate overnight debris from beneath the lens. This might otherwise cause a toxic effect which, when combined with lens adhesion, could precipitate the 'red eye' response [8].

20.1.4 Physical and chemical compatibility of lens materials

The physical aspects of materials must be considered to avoid mechanical trauma from friction or surface hardness. Weight distribution is similarly important. Materials should be chemically inert to avoid surface deposits which could irritate the ocular tissues.

20.2 Approaches to extended wear

On a practical level, extended wear lenses can be divided into three possible groups:

Flexible wear (daily plus)

Many patients requesting extended wear are prepared to accept lenses which they can use safely on an occasional overnight basis, remaining happy to remove them most evenings. This type of lens wear gives maximum flexibility and safety. On a day-to-day basis they are taking advantage of the excellent physiological properties of either high *Dk* hard or high water content soft lenses, while at the same time incurring very little risk of adverse ocular response to occasional overnight use.

Up to 1 week

A maximum of 6 nights' wear followed by 1 night's rest gives a realistic schedule for the majority of patients. Proper lens cleaning and disinfection are maintained by regular removal and a consistent weekly routine is developed. Disposable lenses fit well into such a routine.

Over 1 week

Over 1 week may be regarded as continuous wear or long-term extended wear. It is suitable or even essential for many medical cases, poor lens handlers or for some vocational uses. For most normal eyes, wearing schedules beyond 1 week put additional stress on the cornea and must be used with great caution. There is, however, a small group of experienced patients who have learned a 'sixth sense' of when lenses need removal and encounter fewer problems with handling, breakage, solutions and infections by leaving lenses in the eyes for sometimes several months.

20.3 Patient selection

20.3.1 Indications and contraindications

INDICATIONS

The majority of extended wear lenses are fitted at the patient's request for purely cosmetic reasons. With proper supervision, they generally work well, but there is always the possibility of problems such as infections, oedema or vascularization (*see* Section 20.7). Great care is required not only by the practitioner but also by the patient, who should be made aware of potential hazards. The clinical needs must therefore be carefully balanced against the possible risks.

There are, however, many patients for whom extended wear is the most suitable if not the only possible form of visual correction:

- Aphakics, where handling and visual difficulties preclude daily wear.
- Other poor lens handlers.
- Therapeutic bandage cases (*see* Section 31.4).
- Young children where daily handling is not feasible (*see* Section 29.1).
- Vocations where good vision is required immediately on wakening.
- Where all soft lens disinfection systems create problems.
- Where soft lens patients have no facility for lens disinfection.
- As the rear component of a low vision aid system and handling is impossible.

CONTRAINDICATIONS

- Patients known to be predisposed to corneal oedema.
- Existing corneal vascularization.
- PC.
- Patients unlikely to follow practitioner advice.
- Patients unable to remove lenses.
- Diabetics, where the corneal epithelium is likely to be more fragile.
- Where financial constraints may preclude aftercare and regular lens replacement.

20.3.2 Advantages of soft and hard lenses in extended wear

ADVANTAGES OF SOFT LENSES

- More comfortable.
- Easier adaptation.
- Easier to fit.
- No problems with foreign bodies.
- No 3 and 9 o'clock staining.

ADVANTAGES OF HARD LENSES

- Very high *Dk*s possible.
- Tear pump on blinking.
- Avoidance of trapped debris.
- Reduced risk of infection.
- Better vision.
- Fewer corneal changes.
- Lenses do not cover the entire cornea.
- No lens dehydration.
- Fewer deposit problems.
- Easier lens maintenance.
- No solutions sensitivity.
- Longer life span.

20.4 Soft lens fitting and problems

20.4.1 Fitting

The main consideration is to provide the maximum possible oxygen supply for the cornea. This can be achieved in one of two ways:

- By means of high water content (e.g. Permaflex 74% and Incanto 78%). Lenses have high *Dk* values, but the potential problems are lens fragility, deposits and discolouration, and greater likelihood of solutions reaction.
- By making medium or low water content lenses extremely thin (e.g. Acuvue, 58%; Hydrocurve II, 55%; Bausch and Lomb O Series, 38%; CSI-T, 38%). These rely on good *Dk/t* values but give problems with handling. Hyper-thin lenses also give poor tears exchange on blinking.

Fitting considerations therefore include the following:

- Large refractive errors (both plus and minus) are better fitted with high water content lenses because of average thickness factors.
- Lenses should be as flat as possible consistent with stability of fitting and vision. The exception is the lathed Permalens which is fitted steeper than 'K'.

- Lenses become tighter with wear, particularly overnight because of dehydration.

- Lenses become tighter with age and deposits (*see* Section 28.5).

- Examination during fitting and aftercare must be carried out with the slit lamp, otherwise small degrees of movement cannot be seen.

- Movement should ideally be about 1.00 mm, with a minimum value of 0.50 mm. This ensures proper tears exchange to remove debris from beneath the lens on blinking. It is not always possible with ultra-thin lenses because of the way they drape the cornea.

- Some makes of lens are available only in a limited range of parameters. A compromise fitting should never be accepted with extended wear, since lenses are not removed to allow the resolution of otherwise minor difficulties (e.g. arcuate staining from a decentred lens).

- Some thicker lenses such as aphakics can cause dimpling.

20.4.2 Problems

Lens dehydration and corneal desiccation

Lens dehydration and corneal desiccation can occur with both high water content and ultra-thin low water content lenses. The typical result is punctate staining in the mid-periphery of the cornea in the exposed area of the palpebral aperture. With the more rigid materials it can be associated with superior arcuate staining.

Where there is no obvious fault with the fitting, it is usually necessary to change to another make of lens with different dehydration characteristics [9,10].

'Red eye'

The sudden, acute 'red eye' is a serious and unpredictable complication of soft extended wear giving gross conjunctival hyperaemia. It is usually unilateral, associated with varying degrees of pain, photophobia, lacrimation and limbal infiltrates. The likeliest causes are an inflammatory response to trapped debris and toxins beneath the lens [8,11] and to deposits on the lens surface. The incidence is higher with heat disinfection and reduced with peroxide systems [12].

The courses of action are:

- Remove lenses.
- Ensure patient attends for immediate examination.
- Consider referral.
- Wait several days for condition to resolve.
- Change to new lenses.
- Ensure a peroxide disinfection system is used.
- Consider changing to daily wear – essential if the 'red eye' recurs.

Infections

Infections with extended wear lenses tend to be more severe and longer lasting than with daily wear lenses. Immediate medical treatment is particularly required for corneal ulcers to minimize the risk of permanent visual loss. Other actions are as above for the 'red eye'.

The risks of infection are reduced with:

- Frequent lens replacement.
- Maximum oxygen supply to the cornea.
- Proper lens mobility.
- Proper lens cleaning and maintenance by the patient.
- Hygienic lens handling by the patient.

Papillary conjunctivitis (PC)

The main causes of PC with soft extended wear lenses are deposits and allergic responses during the hay fever season. The incidence is higher with low water content lenses, or where heat disinfection is used with high water content lenses [12]. The courses of action are given in Section 27.3.5.

Oedema

Stromal oedema is the cornea's response to insufficient oxygen under closed eye conditions (see Section 27.3.2) and may show in a variety of ways:

- Single stria, indicating 5–6% swelling.
- Several striae, indicating 7–10% swelling.

- Stromal folds, indicating 10–12% swelling.
- Epithelial microcysts.
- Subjective symptoms of cloudy vision.

Epithelial microcysts

Microcysts contain fluid and cellular debris, appearing as small vesicles in the corneal epithelium, with high magnification on the slit lamp. They represent an indication of hypoxic corneal stress, although small numbers may be considered sufficiently normal to ignore in the absence of other signs. They are generally seen after 2–3 months of extended wear, but can occur sooner [13].

Vascularization

Vascularization is a longer term response of both daily and extended soft lens wear. Vessels may be either superficial, extending from the limbal arcades, or deeper, stromal neovascularization where there is a much greater risk that they may extend into the pupil area. It may be necessary to change from extended to daily wear; from soft to hard lenses; or even, in severe cases, to cease contact lens wear altogether.

Deposits

Because lenses are not removed for cleaning, there is a general predisposition to deposits (*see* Section 28.5). These are kept to a minimum by peroxide and enzyme cleaning and largely avoided with disposable lenses.

Breakage and loss

Most lenses for extended wear are extremely fragile because of thinness or high water content. This is generally acceptable where handling is infrequent, but causes difficulty with more flexible wearing schedules. Loss is not a great problem, although some of the smaller, thinner lenses are occasionally rubbed out of the eye during sleep.

20.5 Hard lens fitting and problems

20.5.1 Fitting

The main considerations are:

- Sufficient oxygen with a high *Dk* material.
- Adequate edge lift to avoid lens adhesion.
- Avoiding excessive edge lift and 3 and 9 o'clock staining.
- Good centration, particularly avoiding low riding lenses because of the risk of adhesion.
- Sufficient lens movement to provide a good tears pump.
- Avoiding lenses which ride onto or over the limbus.

20.5.2 Problems

Overall, there are fewer problems with hard lenses for extended wear. They do not cover the entire cornea, give a regular tear pump and are easier to remove and clean. By their nature, they avoid absorption, solutions reaction, the 'red eye' and vascularization. However, other difficulties can occur, as shown below.

3 and 9 o'clock staining

3 and 9 o'clock staining is the hard lens equivalent of soft lens dehydration. It rarely causes discomfort, but because patients continue to wear lenses its effect may becomes cumulative (*see* Section 27.3.2 for possible remedies).

Infections

Infection with hard lenses is infrequent. Care, however, is required where lens adhesion occurs because of the possibility of corneal ulceration [14,15].

Papillary conjunctivitis

PC can occur with silicone acrylates because of deposits, allergic response or mechanical irritation. It is generally avoided with fluoropolymers.

Oedema

Microcysts and striae occur where materials with insufficient Dk have been used [1].

Vascularization

Vascularization occasionally occurs in the horizontal meridian, associated with prolonged 3 and 9 o'clock staining.

Breakage and loss

Breakage occurs with some of the more brittle high Dk materials and where lenses have crazed or otherwise deteriorated with time. Loss is no worse than with daily wear.

Lens adhesion

Most studies report lens adhesion to the cornea in a minimum of 10% of patients immediately on wakening [14,15]. Sticking relates to lens design, material, lid pressure and changes in tear constituents [16] (*see* Section 27.3.6.). It must be avoided with extended wear because of the risk of corneal ulcers.

20.6 Other lenses for extended wear

20.6.1 Silicone lenses

Silicone lenses (Section 5.4) have extremely high Dks and are occasionally used for extended wear. One of their main applications is with babies to avoid the loss and damage which occur with soft lenses (*see* Section 29.3.1).

20.7 Long-term consequences of extended wear

Metabolic activity

Reduced oxygen supply to the epithelium reduces metabolic rate and therefore cell mitosis. Since the epithelium would not remain intact with decreased cell production and a constant rate of cell death and removal at the anterior epithelial surface, some compensation must occur.

Infection

The chances of infection, including microbial keratitis and sterile infiltrates, are significantly greater if the cells at the anterior epithelial surface become functionally less resistant as a result of long-term extended wear [17].

Corneal thinning

Epithelial thinning occurs as cell production and wastage rates reach a new equilibrium. Stromal thinning results from long-term chronic oedema [4].

Endothelial polymegathism

Polymegathism is an irregularity in the cell size of the corneal endothelium caused by a lowering of pH [18] due to increased lactic acid (resulting from lens-induced hypoxia) [19] and/or increased carbonic acid (resulting from lens-induced hypercapnia). There does not seem to be a change in cell density, but a size increase of 27% has been reported [4]. The chances of complications with surgery or trauma are reported to be significantly greater after extended wear [20].

Vascularization

The extension of limbal blood vessels into the cornea is a serious indication of chronic hypoxia. The vessels may extend from any position around the limbus, but tend to be further advanced beneath the top lid. Any increase should be monitored and if the vessels grow more than 2 mm into the cornea extended wear should be discontinued.

Neovascularization

New vessel growth at a deep stromal level is an unacceptable response to corneal stress caused by hypoxia, limbal compression or tissue damage. If allowed to continue and encroach within the pupil area, vision may be reduced as the surrounding tissue is changed by a lipid keratopathy.

Practical advice

To minimize the risk of potential problems, both short- and long-term patients should:

- Return for regular aftercare visits, not only during the fitting stage but for as long as extended wear continues.
- Replace lenses on a routine basis, at least every 12 months.
- Use peroxide and enzyme systems.
- Receive written instructions.
- Receive advice that they *must* remove lenses if they suffer:

  red eyes,
  discomfort,
  reduced vision,
  persistent lacrimation,
  other abnormal symptoms,
  illness.

References

1. Holden, B.A. and Mertz, G.W. (1984) Critical oxygen levels to avoid corneal oedema for daily and extended wear contact lenses. *Investigative Ophthalmology and Visual Science*, **25**, 1161
2. Holden, B.A. and Sweeney, D.F. (1987) Ocular requirements for extended wear. *Contax*, May, 13–18
3. Holden, B.A., Sweeney, D.F. and Sanderson, G. (1984) The minimum precorneal oxygen tension to avoid corneal oedema. *Investigative Ophthalmology and Visual Science*, **25**, 476
4. Holden, B.A., Sweeney, D.F., Vannas, A., Nilsson, K.T. and Efron, N. (1985) Effects of long-term extended contact lens wear on the human cornea. *Investigative Ophthalmology and Visual Science*, **26**, 1489
5. Hamano, H., Hori, M., Hamano, T., Kawabe, H., Mikami, M., Mitsunaga, S. et al. (1983) Effects of contact lens wear on mitosis of corneal epithelium and lactate content of aqueous humor of rabbit. *Japanese Journal of Ophthalmology*, **27**, 451
6. Madigan, M.C., Holden, B.A. and Kwok, L.S. (1986) Extended wear of hydrogel contact lenses can compromise the corneal epithelium. *Investigative Ophthalmology and Visual Science*, **27** (suppl.), 140
7. Millodot, M. (1976) Effect of the length of wear of contact lenses on corneal sensitivity. *Acta Ophthalmologica*, **54**, 721
8. Josephson, J.E. and Caffrey, B.E. (1979) Infiltrative keratitis in hydrogel wearers. *International Contact Lens Clinic*, **6**, 223–242
9. Holden, B.A. (1986) Epithelial erosions caused by thin high water contact lenses. *Clinical and Experimental Optometry*, **69**, 103–107
10. Gasson, A.P. (1987) Aftercare problems with extended wear lenses. *Optician*, **193**(5078), 15–19

11. Zantos, S.G. and Holden, B.A. (1978) Ocular changes associated with continuous wear of contact lenses. *Australian Journal of Optometry*, **61**, 418–426

12. Kotow, M., Grant, T. and Holden, B.A. (1986) Evaluation of current care and maintenance systems for hydrogel extended wear. *Transactions of the British Contact Lens Association Annual Clinical Conference*, **3**, 66–67

13. Zantos, S. (1983) Cystic formations in the corneal epithelium during extended wear of contact lenses. *International Contact Lens Clinic*, **10**, 128–146

14. Zabkewicz, K., Swarbrick, H. and Holden, B.A. (1986) Clinical experience with low to moderate *Dk* hard gas permeable lenses for extended wear. *Transactions of the British Contact Lens Association Annual Clinical Conference*, **3**, 101–102

15. Swarbrick, H.A. and Holden, B.A. (1989) Rigid gas-permeable lens binding: significance and contributing factors. *American Journal of Optometry and Physiological Optics*, **64**, 815–823

16. Polse, K.A., Rivera, R.K. and Bonanno, J.A. (1988) Ocular effects of hard gas permeable lens extended wear. *American Journal of Optometry and Physiological Optics*, **65**, 358–364

17. Stapleton, F., Dart, J and Minassian, D. (1989) Contact lens related infiltrates – risk figures for different lens types and association with lens hygiene and solution contamination. *Transactions of the British Contact Lens Association Annual Clinical Conference*, **6**, 52–55

18. Bonanno, J.A. and Polse, K.A. (1987) Measurement of *in vivo* human corneal stroma pH: open and closed eyes. *Investigative Ophthalmology and Visual Science*, **28**, 522–530

19. Holden, B.A., Ross, R. and Jenkins, J. (1987) Hydrogel contact lenses impede carbon dioxide efflux from the human cornea. *Current Eye Research*, **6**, 1283–1290

20. Rao, G.N., Aquavella, J.V., Goldberg, S.H. and Berk, S.L. (1984) Pseudo aphakic bullous keratopathy – relationship to preoperative corneal endothelial status *Ophthalmology*, **91**, 1135

Chapter 21

Toric hard lenses

21.1 Patient selection

21.1.1 Indications and contraindications

INDICATIONS

To improve the physical fit

- The difference between principal meridians is greater than 0.6 mm.
- A spherical lens is unstable.
- A spherical lens decentres.
- A spherical lens gives unacceptable bearing areas due to the corneal toricity.
- The bearing areas minimize tears exchange.
- A spherical lens produces corneal moulding and unacceptable spectacle blur.
- The cornea becomes significantly more toric towards the periphery.

To give optimum visual acuity

- Residual astigmatism is greater than about 1.00 D.
- Induced astigmatism.

CONTRAINDICATIONS

- Where a spherical lens gives a satisfactory result.
- Sensitive eyes where increased thickness causes discomfort or reduces transmissibility to an unacceptable level.
- Critical visual needs where visual acuity may be unstable.
- With a toric cornea but spherical spectacle Rx (*see* Section 3.4).
- The greater expense of toric lenses.

● A toric lens is unnecessary with an amblyopic eye.

21.1.2 Residual and induced astigmatism

Residual astigmatism

Residual astigmatism is the uncorrected astigmatism found by refraction when a spherical contact lens is placed on the cornea. It derives from the crystalline lens and is usually against-the-rule. It is predictable where the spectacle cylinder and 'K' readings do not correlate. The corneal astigmatism is neutralized by a hard lens leaving the lenticular astigmatism uncorrected.

Example 1:

Spectacle Rx: $-3.00/-1.50 \times 95$ 'K' 7.90 mm × 7.85 mm
Corneal astigmatism $= 0.05$ mm $\equiv 0.25$ D
Residual astigmatism $= 1.25$ D

Example 2:

Spectacle Rx: $-2.00/-1.00 \times 180$ 'K' 7.60 mm (along 180°)
                                                     7.80 mm (along 90°)
Corneal astigmatism $= 0.20$ mm $\equiv 1.00$ D
Residual astigmatism $= 2.00$ D

Induced astigmatism

The liquid lens beneath a hard contact lens neutralizes only 9/10 of the anterior corneal astigmatism because of the difference in refractive indices [1].

Induced astigmatism is created when a toric back surface is placed on a toric cornea. It occurs because of the different refractive indices of the lens material and the tears. The induced astigmatism is against-the-rule if the corneal and spectacle astigmatism is with-the-rule.

21.2 Lens designs

There are six possible designs for the correction of astigmatism of which four are toroidal.

21.2.1 Non-toric lens forms

Small spherical lenses

Lenses with very small TDs are often successful. They fit only the central area of the cornea which may be more spherical than the periphery. Fitting sets with narrow axial edge lift (typically 0.10 mm) are used to avoid excessive edge clearance or stand-off in the steeper meridian.

Practical advice

- Lenses may sometimes be as small as 7.50 mm.
- Centration is important to avoid flare.
- Use a centre thickness in the region of 0.12 mm.

Aspheric lenses

Most aspheric designs also have narrow edge lift and give reduced clearances along the steeper meridian. In some cases they can mask up to about 4.00 D of astigmatism. They are usually fitted in alignment or flatter to avoid flexure.

21.2.2 Toric lenses

Front surface toric

A spherical back surface with a front surface cylinder to correct *residual astigmatism*. Stabilization is necessary to maintain the correct cylinder axis.

Toric periphery

A spherical BOZR with toric back peripheral radii. Used to give stability and fit corneas where peripheral toricity is significantly greater than central. The front surface is usually spherical.

Back surface toric

Both central and peripheral radii are toric with a spherical front surface. The final peripheral radius is sometimes spherical for ease of manufacture and to assist tear flow. Stabilization should be unnecessary, since the lens radii should correctly follow the principal meridians of the cornea.

Bitoric lenses

Both central and peripheral back surface radii are toric, combined with a front surface cylinder to correct *induced astigmatism*.

Stabilization is usually needed for correct orientation of the cylinder axis because its position is important.

21.3 Methods of stabilization

PRISM BALLAST

Prism ballast usually employs $1.5^\triangle$, with an upper limit of about $3^\triangle$. The prism base should always orientate downwards and be marked to assist observation. The stabilizing effect of gravity on the thicker lower edge is also helped by lid action.

TRUNCATION

Truncation may be used either on its own or in conjunction with prism ballast and can be single or double. A chord of 0.50–1.00 mm is removed from the lens edge and the optimum effect is achieved when the truncation sits on the lower lid. It is therefore ineffective with small diameters. To assist stability, the TD of the optimum trial lens should be increased by 0.50 mm for single truncation and up to 1 mm for double.

21.4 Fitting front surface torics

Method 1

- Use a large spherical trial lens with power as near as possible to the final Rx and over-refract to find the maximum minus sphere.
- Order a lens based on this power, usually with $1.5^\triangle$.
- Always have the prism base marked so that the lens orientation can be measured on the eye.
- Over-refract and record the cylinder in *positive* form.
- Note the orientation of the prism base.
- If the lens is unstable, consider a truncation of 0.50 mm, increasing the prism or a larger TD.
- Order the front cylinder in *positive* form, taking into account any rotation of the lens.
- The cylinder can be worked on the initial lens if no other changes are needed.

Method 2

- Over-refract with a spherical trial lens and order the final prescription lens directly with the front surface cylinder.
- This procedure is quicker, but an estimate of the final lens orientation is required (usually 5–15° nasal).

Practical advice

- If only one eye requires a front toric, there may be problems with tolerance.
- Use truncation if there is a problem with binocular vision because of prism in only one eye.

Example
'K' readings: 7.55 mm × 7.45 mm
Spectacle *Rx*:   −2.75/−1.50 × 80
C3 Tor FS 7.50:7.00/8.10:8.00/10.75:9.90
    BVP −4.00/+0.75 × 170   1.5$^\triangle$ base 280
    Mark one dot on the prism base the and another on the apex
    Lower truncation. Remove 0.50 mm along 180°

21.5 Fitting toric peripheries

- A toric periphery with a spherical BOZR gives an oval optic with the smallest diameter along the flatter meridian.
- A toric periphery trial set should ideally be used, looking for a regular fluorescein pattern in the periphery.
- Trial sets usually have TDs of 8.50–9.50 mm and relatively small BOZDs of 6.50–7.00 mm.
- With a spherical trial set, the fitting should be assessed for central alignment and correct peripheral clearance in the flatter meridian.
- The radius for the steeper peripheral meridian can be determined either from the 'K' readings or the fluorescein pattern. A minimum toric difference of 0.60 mm is usually required.
- The secondary curves are approximately 0.80–1.20 mm flatter.

● The final curve may be spherical.

Examples
'K'   7.90 mm × 7.50 mm
    C3 7.90:7.00/8.90:8.20/11.30:9.00
              8.30   10.70
    C3 7.90:7.00/8.90:8.20/10.75:9.00
              8.30

ADVANTAGES

● Ideal for corneas which become more toric towards the periphery.
● Good acuity, since the liquid lens neutralizes the corneal astigmatism.
● Fairly easy to manufacture.
● Less expensive than full back surface toric lenses.

DISADVANTAGES

● They are a compromise fit.
● They can rotate more than a full back surface toric and may cause corneal insult.

21.6 Fitting back surface torics

21.6.1 Toric fitting set

● A trial lens is selected to have the flatter meridian the same as flattest 'K' and the steeper meridian 0.1 mm flatter than steepest 'K'. The meridians are therefore not exactly matched (e.g. 'K' 8.00 × 7.40; BOZR 8.00 × 7.50).
● The ideal fluorescein pattern should look the same as an alignment spherical fit.
● Over-refraction should be carried out with *minus* cylinders. The spherical component is the power along the flattest meridian.
● The laboratory will produce the cylinder along the steeper meridian.
● The possibility of induced astigmatism must always be considered.

21.6.2 Spherical fitting set

- A spherical lens is fitted in alignment to establish the flatter meridian.
- The steeper radius is determined from the 'K' readings.
- The spherical power is determined by over-refraction with *minus* cylinders.
- The cylinder is obtained by calculation.

Example
Ocular refraction: −2.00/−3.00 × 180
Keratometry: 8.00 mm along 180°; 7.45 mm along 90°
The astigmatism is entirely corneal.
Trial lens radius giving alignment along 180° = 8.00 mm
By fluorescein assessment toric lens needed is: r_{01} = 8.00 along 180° and r_{02} = 7.55 along 90°
BVP calculation:
Along 180° BVP = −2.00 D (from over-refraction with trial lens)
Along 90°   BOZR of 7.55 gives anterior surface power to the tear lens in air of (refractive index of tears n = 1.336):

$$F = \frac{n-1}{r_0}$$

$$\frac{336}{7.55} = +44.50$$

BOZR of 8.00 gives anterior surface power to the tear lens in air of:

$$\frac{336}{8.00} = +42.00$$

Tear lens anterior surface astigmatism = −2.50 D
Final prescription is:
TBS $\underline{8.00}$:7.00/$\underline{8.60}$:8.00/$\underline{10.50}$:9.00
    7.55   8.15   10.00
    −2.00/−2.50 × 180

The rule of thumb, 0.1 mm ≡ 0.50 D, gives useful confirmation, since 8.00 mm − 7.55 mm is 0.45 mm ≡ 2.25 D.

21.6.3 Fitting by calculation

A lens can also be ordered for the patient by theoretical calculation using the ocular refraction, 'K' readings and refractive index of the material. BOZD, TD and edge clearance are nevertheless determined from clinical assessment. The toric difference of the lens radii can be chosen to neutralize the corneal astigmatism, but the induced astigmatism must also be calculated.

Example

$$\frac{1.336 - 1.480}{r_{01}} - \frac{1.336 - 1.480}{r_{02}}$$

where
1.336 = refractive index (RI) of tears
1.480 = refractive index of typical silicone/acrylate material
r_{01} = steeper radius of curvature, in metres
r_{02} = flatter radius of curvature, in metres

Hence, induced astigmatism

$$= \frac{-144}{r_{01}} - \frac{-144}{r_{02}} \quad r_{01} \text{ and } r_{02} \text{ in mm}$$

Rule of thumb

Choosing the lens radii to be approximately 75% of the corneal toric difference often avoids a bitoric lens.

Lenticular astigmatism is assumed where the ocular astigmatism is greater than that found with the keratometer. This is sometimes effectively neutralized by the induced astigmatism without the need for a front surface cylinder.

Example

Spectacle prescription $-2.00/-3.00 \times 180$
    Keratometry   8.00 mm along 180°; 7.60 mm along 90°
    Corneal astigmatism 0.40 mm = -2.00 D
    Residual astigmatism $(-3.00) - (-2.00) = -1.00$ D
    BOZRs chosen $r_{01} = 7.70$ mm; $r_{02} = 8.00$ mm

From above: induced astigmatism $= \dfrac{-144}{7.70} - \dfrac{-144}{8.00}$

    Induced astigmatism $(-18.70) - (-18.00) = -0.70$ D

This almost exactly corrects the residual astigmatism and a front surface cylinder is unnecessary.

The final power of the steeper meridian can be determined by calculation, but it is often better left to the laboratory:

$$\frac{1 - 1.480}{7.70} - \frac{1 - 1.480}{8.00} = (-62.33) - (-60.00) = -2.33$$

As induced cylinder is neutralized the final powers are:

BVP along flatter meridian $= -2.00$
BVP along steeper $= -2.00 + (-2.33) = -4.33$
                   $-2.00/-2.33$ along flatter meridian

DISADVANTAGES

● If corneal and ocular astigmatism are equal, induced astigmatism is created and may require correction.

● If the ocular astigmatism is less than the corneal astigmatism, lenticular astigmatism is revealed by a hard lens and requires neutralizing together with the induced astigmatism. In this case, a large front surface cylinder is needed.

21.7 Fitting bitorics

A bitoric is required when a back surface toric has created sufficient induced astigmatism (usually over 0.75 D) to warrant correction with a front surface cylinder. Fitting is carried out as described in Section 21.6.

A further calculation is required to determine the final back vertex power in air [2]:

Example
The ocular refraction has a sphere S and a cylinder C.
The lens has $n = 1.480$ and radii r_{01} and r_{02}.
The astigmatism induced by the back surface in air A is given by:

$$A = \frac{1 - 1.480}{r_{01}} - \frac{1 - 1.480}{r_{02}}$$

$$= \frac{-480}{r_{01}} - \frac{-480}{r_{02}}$$

If the corneal and ocular astigmatism are equal, the BVP along the flatter meridian is S.

The power along the steeper meridian is $S + A$

To correct the induced astigmatism, I, this becomes $S + A - I$

Thus the BVP of a lens is:
  S along the flatter
  $S + A - I$ along the steeper

Example

Spectacle prescription	$-2.00/-3.00 \times 180$
Keratometry	8.00 mm along 180°; 7.40 mm along 90°
Corneal astigmatism	3.00 D
Residual astigmatism	0.00 D

From fitting (*see* Section 21.6.1) $r_1 = 7.50$ mm; $r_2 = 8.00$ mm

$$\text{Induced astigmatism } \frac{-144}{7.50} - \frac{-144}{8.00}$$

$$(-19.20) - (-18.00) = -1.20\,\text{D}$$

This degree of induced astigmatism requires correction.

The astigmatism induced by the back surface in air:

$$\frac{-480}{7.50} - \frac{-480}{8.00} = (-64.00) - (-60.00) = -4.00$$

BVP along flatter meridian $= -2.00\,\text{D}$
BVP along steeper meridian $= (-2.00) + (-4.00) - (-1.20)$
$$= -4.80\,\text{D}$$

Equivalent to $-2.00/-2.80$ along flatter meridian

Reference

1. Douthwaite, W.A. (1987) *Contact Lens Optics*, Butterworth-Heinemann, Oxford.
2. Edwards, K.H. (1982) The calculation and fitting of toric lenses. *Ophthalmic Optician*, **22**, 106–114

Chapter 22

Toric soft lenses

22.1 Patient selection

Toric soft lenses are not prescribed to improve the physical fitting, as with hard lenses (except with very high degrees of astigmatism), but to provide good visual acuity where spherical lenses are unable to achieve this.

INDICATIONS

- Vision is unsatisfactory with a spherical soft lens.
- Astigmatism is 1.00 D or greater (occasionally 0.75 D or 0.50 D cylinders may be fitted).
- Tolerance is poor with a hard lens.
- Keratometry and optical considerations indicate that a hard lens requires a much more complex, bitoric design (*see* Section 21.7).

CONTRAINDICATIONS

- Astigmatism is purely corneal and hard lens tolerance is good.
- Existing hard lens wearers.
- Irregular astigmatism.
- Monocular patients.

22.2 Stabilization

22.2.1 Influences on lens behaviour

The main influences on lens orientation are method of stabilization and the lids. Eyelids are important in respect of:

- Position of lower lid.

- Size of vertical palpebral aperture.
- Lid tension.
- Force of blink.
- Direction of movement on blinking.

In cases of with-the-rule astigmatism, the thickest portions of the correcting toric lie at the top and bottom of the lens. The normal action of the lids is to rotate the lens 90° off-axis to bring the thickest parts into the horizontal meridian. The action of the lids on the lens edge has been compared to squeezing a water melon seed, so that they control the ultimate lens position even with the head inverted [1].

There are several other factors which have some effect on lens behaviour [2]:

- Gravity.
- Water content.
- Material elasticity.
- Lens thickness.
- Hydrostatic pressure.

22.2.2 Methods of stabilization

Various techniques are possible, either on their own or in combination.

TRUNCATION

Truncation is usually single, removing a 1 mm chord from the lower edge of the lens at right-angles to the base–apex line. Oblique truncations (up to 20°) are feasible and sometimes used with angled lids. Some designs of front surface toric employ double truncation.

Advantages

- Better stability than other methods.
- Easily observed and measured on the eye.
- Thinner lenses can be used.

Disadvantages

- Less comfortable.

- Buckling of lower edge if too flat or vertical corneal meridian very steep.
- Cosmetically more noticeable.
- Less satisfactory with oblique cylinders.
- Increased deposits along truncated edge.

PRISM BALLAST

Prism ballast usually employs $1^\triangle$ or $1.5^\triangle$ base down. The upper limit is approximately $3^\triangle$. Two modern refinements of lens design are able to reduce the thickness previously associated with this method and give improved comfort and physiological response:

- Prism-free optics to incorporate the stabilizing prism only in the peripheral areas of the lens (e.g. Hydron Z6 toric).
- Slab-off prisms to give equal thickness at both the base and 3 and 9 o'clock positions.

Where a toric is required for only one eye, in theory the spherical lens for the other eye should also include base-down prism to prevent binocular imbalance. This is not often necessary in practice (not at all with prism-free optics) and the spherical lens is usually ordered without prism but with subsequent assessment of binocularity.

Advantages

- More comfortable than truncation.
- Better with oblique cylinders.
- Cosmetically less noticeable.

Disadvantages

- Careful slit-lamp observation required to assess lens orientation.
- Lenses are thicker.
- Greater risk of oedema with low water content.

THIN ZONES (DYNAMIC STABILIZATION)

Top and bottom portions of the lens are chamfered to reduce the thickness where the stabilization zones fit beneath the lids

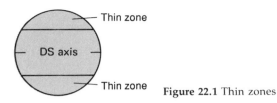

Figure 22.1 Thin zones

(Figure 22.1). The optic portion is the central band which lies within the palpebral aperture. Lenses have the 'DS axis' marked in the 3 and 9 o'clock positions.

Advantages

- Lens remains thin overall.
- Good comfort with thin edges.
- Good cosmetic appearance.

Disadvantages

- Careful slit-lamp observation required to assess lens orientation.
- Limitation to the amount of cylinder (approximately 4.00 D).

TORIC BACK SURFACE

A toric back surface has a natural stabilizing effect when placed in apposition to an equivalently toroidal cornea because least elastic distortion occurs when the lens is correctly aligned. A better result, however, is achieved when used in conjunction with prism ballast or truncation. The toroidal optic zone is ellipsoidal in shape, the dimensions depending upon power and radius. It is larger with a lower cylinder and vice versa.

OTHER METHODS

- Lens elevations (orientation cams) in the 3 and 9 o'clock positions (e.g. Lunelle, Weflex 55).
- Specially shaped, non-circular lenses.

22.2.3 Assessing lens rotation

LENS MARKINGS

In order to assess any rotation on the eye, it is essential that lenses are marked with reference points except for truncations which are easily measureable. The following methods are commonly used:

- A single dot usually at the base of the prism although occasionally at the apex (e.g. Weflex 55).
- Radial engravings at the base of the prism. These are usually separated by 15° (e.g. Z6T) or 30° (e.g. Hydrocurve II) to give a measurement of rotation on the eye (Figure 22.2).
- Horizontal lines in the 3 and 9 o'clock positions (e.g. Torisoft, Hydroflex-m-T) (Figure 22.3).
- Horizontal elevations in the 3 and 9 o'clock positions (e.g. Lunelle).

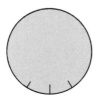

Figure 22.2 Radial engravings

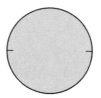

Figure 22.3 Laser lines at 3 and 9 o'clock positions

MEASURING LENS ROTATION

Apart from truncations, engravings can only be clearly observed with the slit lamp. Rotation can be measured by:

- Assessing radial markings by observation alone.
- A graticule, either internal or surrounding the slit lamp eyepiece.
- Rotating a fine slit lamp beam to align with lens engravings and reading the instrument's external protractor scale. Horizontal markings tend to be easier to assess than vertical.
- Using a Javal-type ophthalmometer [3].

22.3 Lens designs

Several different designs have evolved so that toric soft lenses, apart from stabilization with any of the methods in Section

22.2.2, may be of either corneal or semi-scleral diameter; use a variety of water contents; and have either a front or back toric surface.

TOTAL DIAMETER

Advantages of corneal diameter torics (e.g. Hydroflex/m-T)

● Less risk of oedema.
● Cosmetically better.
● Less lower lid sensation.

Advantages of semi-scleral torics (e.g. Hydron Z6T, Weicon T)

● Better stability.
● Less upper lid sensation.
● Wider range of lenses and methods of stabilization.

WATER CONTENT

Advantages of low water content torics (e.g. Hydroflex-TS, Optima)

● Better stability on the eye.
● More reliable orientation.
● Can be made thinner.
● More reproducible.
● Longer life span.
● Easier to manufacture.
● Wider range of lenses available.

Advantages of high water content torics (e.g. Lunelle)

● Better comfort.
● Less risk of oedema.

FRONT AND BACK SURFACE TORICS

Front surface torics

Front surface torics are capable of correcting both corneal and lenticular astigmatism, up to about 4.50 D. They are successful with a wide variety of geometries, both corneal (e.g. Hydroflex

AT, Hoya) and semi-scleral (e.g. Weicon T). Stabilization can be by means of prism ballast (e.g. Optima); truncation (e.g. Hydron *Rx* toric); or dynamic stabilization (e.g. Torisoft, Hanita). The back surface may be either spherical (e.g. Weflex) or aspheric (e.g. Hydron *Rx* toric).

Back surface torics

Back surface torics have evolved logically from the fact that most of the astigmatism encountered in practice is predominantly corneal. Keratometry and spectacle *Rx* give an immediate prediction of the likelihood of visual success. The back surface of the lens is essentially designed to neutralize the toric cornea by replacing it with a spherical front surface. The radii of the principal meridians may be either predetermined by the laboratory (e.g. Hydrocurve II 55) or individually calculated (e.g. Hydroflex/m-T) using a radius to surface power conversion chart (Table 22.1). Cylinders as high as 6.00 D can be corrected. Lenticular astigmatism is not theoretically correctable, although in practice reasonable clinical results can sometimes be obtained. The back surface is sometimes stable enough on its own, but is markedly assisted by either prism ballast (e.g. Durasoft 2) or truncation (e.g. Hydroflex TS).

Table 22.1 Radius to surface power conversion for $n = 1.4448$

BCOR (mm)	Surface power (D)	BCOR (mm)	Surface power (D)
6.00	74.13	8.00	55.60
6.10	72.92	8.10	54.91
6.20	71.74	8.20	54.24
6.30	70.60	8.30	53.59
6.40	69.50	8.40	52.95
6.50	68.43	8.50	52.33
6.60	67.39	8.60	51.72
6.70	66.39	8.70	51.13
6.80	65.41	8.80	50.55
6.90	64.46	8.90	49.98
7.00	63.54	9.00	49.42
7.10	62.65	9.10	48.88
7.20	61.78	9.20	48.35
7.30	60.93	9.30	47.83
7.40	60.11	9.40	47.32
7.50	59.31	9.50	46.82
7.60	58.53	9.60	46.33
7.70	57.77	9.70	45.86
7.80	57.03	9.80	45.39
7.90	56.30	9.90	44.93

22.4 Fitting

Lenses may either be individually designed and prescribed or selected from a simplified range of parameters predetermined by the laboratory (stock torics).

Individually designed lenses

The design method permits the fitting of most prescriptions which it is technically feasible to manufacture, with a comprehensive range of lens parameters, water contents, spherical and cylinder powers, axis positions, and methods of stabilization. The main disadvantages are the length of time required to obtain lenses and additional costs, particularly where changes to the prescription are necessary.

Stock torics

The simplified method enables rapid fitting from either practitioner or laboratory stock, since parameters are carefully restricted. Cylinder powers have an upper range of about 2.50 D (this will cope with 90% of prescriptions [4]), and may be limited to 0.50 D or 0.75 D steps. Axes may be restricted to 20° either side of horizontal or vertical in 10° steps, and oblique cylinders, which are generally more difficult to fit, are frequently omitted.

No single make of standard design, even in the common range of astigmatism, can approach the accuracy of a properly calculated practitioner specification. However, by using several makes of stock toric, a standard design can usually be found to match the correction and fitting required. This is then the preferred method of fitting.

FITTING ROUTINE

- Assess spectacle *Rx* and 'K' readings.
- Decide on a back or front surface toric in respect of corneal or lenticular astigmatism.
- Decide on method of stabilization. A different design placed on each eye usually determines both a preference in comfort by the patient and establishes whether prism, dynamic stabilization or truncation is likely to give best orientation.
- Determine the best fitting trial lens.
- Determine the lens orientation on the eye from the angle at

which the truncation settles or from the markings present on most non-truncated lenses. Trial lenses establish at the fitting stage whether compensation is required for the cylinder axis. The most common result is a 5° nasal rotation of the lens base. Success is unlikely if the rotation is more than about 20°, even if consistent, and it is usually better to try a different fitting or lens type. Oblique cylinders generally give less reliable results.

● Over-refract with a fully settled spherical trial lens of power as near as possible to the spectacle *Rx*. Apart from any vertex distance considerations, this is always worthwhile to ensure that the results correlate, particularly in respect of cylinder power and axis. If there is any discrepancy, repeat with a different trial lens.

● There is little value in over-refracting with a toric trial lens, since the result will be that of obliquely crossed cylinders and

Table 22.2 Residual refractive error induced by mislocation of toric lenses of various cylindrical powers (From Holden and Frauenhofer [4], with permission)

Convention	(1) Axes in standard axis notation (2) Anti-clockwise is +ve, clockwise −ve	
Mislocation (degrees)	$-1.00\,D$	$-2.00\,D\ (\times 2)$
5	$+0.08/-0.16 \times 42.5$	$+0.17/-0.34 \times 42.5$
10	$+0.17/-0.34 \times 40$	$+0.35/-0.69 \times 40$
15	$+0.26/-0.52 \times 37.5$	$+0.52/-1.04 \times 37.5$
20	$+0.34/-0.69 \times 35$	$+0.68/-1.37 \times 35$
25	$+0.43/-0.85 \times 32.5$	$+0.85/-1.69 \times 32.5$
30	$+0.50/-1.00 \times 30$	$+1.00/-2.00 \times 30$
35	$+0.57/-1.14 \times 27.5$	$+1.14/-2.29 \times 27.5$
40	$+0.64/-1.28 \times 25$	$+1.29/-2.57 \times 25$
45	$+0.71/-1.42 \times 22.5$	$+1.41/-2.83 \times 22.5$
50	$+0.76/-1.53 \times 20$	$+1.53/-3.06 \times 20$
55	$+0.82/-1.64 \times 17.5$	$+1.64/-3.28 \times 17.5$
60	$+0.87/-1.73 \times 15$	$+1.73/-3.46 \times 15$
65	$+0.90/-1.82 \times 12.5$	$+1.81/-3.63 \times 12.5$
70	$+0.94/-1.88 \times 10$	$+1.88/-3.76 \times 10$
75	$+0.96/-1.93 \times 7.5$	$+1.93/-3.85 \times 7.5$
80	$+0.98/-1.97 \times 5$	$+1.97/-3.94 \times 5$
85	$+0.99/-1.99 \times 2.5$	$+1.99/-3.98 \times 2.5$
90	$+1.00/-2.00 \times 180$	$+2.00/-4.00 \times 180$

only indirect information may be gained. (see Table 22.2) However, the dynamics of a toric lens on the eye are likely to be more reliable than a spherical lens because a correcting cylinder has been incorporated.

- If axis compensation has been made because of lens rotation at the initial fitting, the prescription lens should also settle with exactly the same degree of rotation.

- The nature of the over-refraction may be used as a guide with the toric prescription lens, although its absolute value is not very meaningful. If cylinder is present at the original axis or at 90° to this, under- or over-correction is suggested. If it takes the form of a plus sphere with minus cylinder of approximately twice the power (e.g. +0.50−1.00) at a different axis, it is because of cylinder axis mislocation. This may be due to lens rotation or inaccurate manufacture and may be assessed from Table 22.2.

22.5 Fitting examples

Example 1

FRONT SURFACE STOCK TORIC

Spectacle Rx: R.E. −3.00/−1.25 × 85

Keratometry. R.E. 7.85 mm (43.00 D) spherical

The astigmatism is entirely lenticular, so a front surface toric is required.

Best fitting: Ciba, Torisoft 8.90:14.50   −3.00

Over-refraction: Plano/−1.25 × 85

Trial lens: Locates with 5° nasal (anti-clockwise) rotation.

The nearest options available for this stock design are:

Cylinders: −1.00 D or −1.75 D. It is nearly always better to under- rather than over-correct. Select −1.00 D.

Axes: 80° or 90°. Select 80° because of the 5° nasal orientation of the trial lens. The cylinder axis will therefore rotate to the required 85°.

Lens specification: 8.90:14.50   −3.00/−1.00 × 80

Example 2

FRONT SURFACE TORIC WITH FULL RANGE OF PARAMETERS

Spectacle Rx: L.E. −2.50/−3.50 × 180

Keratometry: L.E. 8.23 mm along 180° (41.00 D)
                     7.72 mm along 90° (43.75 D)

The astigmatism is outside the range of a stock toric. Most is corneal but with 0.75 D lenticular. Select a front surface toric with a full range of parameters.

Best fitting: Hydron Z6 Toric   9.00:14.00   −3.00

Over-refraction: +0.50/−3.25 × 180

Lens specification allowing for 5° nasal (clockwise) rotation: 9.00:14.00 − 2.50/−3.25 × 5

Suppose this prescription lens proved too mobile and also settled consistently with 10° temporal (anti-clockwise) rotation. Re-order:

Final lens specification: 8.70:14.00   −2.50/−3.25 × 170

Example 3

BACK SURFACE TORIC

Spectacle Rx: R.E. −1.25 DS/−2.50 DC × 20

Keratometry: R.E. 7.96 mm along 20° (42.50 D)
                     7.50 mm along 110° (45.00 D)

The astigmatism is entirely corneal and possibly within the range of a stock toric.

Best fitting: Hydrocurve II 55   8.80:14.50   −1.50

Example 3A

Over-refraction: +0.25/−2.25 × 20

Trial lens: Locates with 5° nasal (anti-clockwise) rotation.

Lens specification: 8.80:14.50   −1.25/−2.00 × 15

Example 3B

Over-refraction: Plano/−2.75 × 25

Trial lens: Locates with 20° temporal (clockwise) rotation.

With 0.75 D under-correction of the cylinder and a required axis theoretically at an oblique 45°, this example is unlikely to give a successful result. Discontinue and try another variety of toric, probably with truncation for better stability.

Example 4

BACK SURFACE TORIC FITTED BY CALCULATION

Spectacle Rx: R.E. −0.75/−3.50 × 15

Keratometry: R.E. 8.23 mm along 15 (41.00 D)
7.63 mm along 105 (44.25 D)

The astigmatism is almost entirely corneal and outside the range of a stock toric. Suppose non-truncated designs give unstable and excessive rotation. Select a back surface toric with truncation.

Best fitting: Hydroflex TS   9.30:14.00   −3.00

Over-refraction: +2.50/−3.50 × 15
(N.B. This is required in minus cylinder form. There is also the typical +0.25 D difference in spherical power due to liquid lens and flexure effects − *see* Chapter 17.)

Trial lens: Locates with 10° nasal rotation. Prescription lens therefore requires a compensated axis at 5° (designated T5)

Calculation of radii for principal meridians

The trial lens radius is taken as the flatter meridian and, using Table 22.1, converted to surface power (N.B. minus sign).

9.30 mm   →   −47.83 D   surface power
           add   −3.50 D   correcting cylinder

8.70 mm   ←   −51.33 D

The nearest value to 51.33 D in Table 22.1 is 51.13 D (8.70 mm) and is taken as the steeper meridian.

Final lens specification: 9.30/8.70:14.00   −0.50   T5

N.B. If the prescription lens over-corrects the astigmatism, this is possibly due to induced astigmatism and a smaller toric difference is indicated.

Practical advice

- A successul fitting usually returns consistently to the same orientation within one or two blinks.
- Where a lens mislocates on the eye, rather than attempt to change its orientation (e.g. by tightening the fit or adjusting the truncation), assume that the various stabilizing factors (*see* Section 22.2.1) will always act on the lens in a similar way. Compensate in the axis of the correcting cylinder for any lens rotation on the eye.
- Fitting is more difficult with oblique cylinders.
- Take particular care when fitting essentially monocular patients. They are much more disturbed by any instability of vision caused by temporary lens rotation on blinking.
- If no success is achieved after the second lens for a particular eye, try a different type of design.

References

1. Killpartrick, M.R. (1983) Apples, space-time and the watermelon seed. *Ophthalmic Optician*, **23**, 801–802
2. Grant, R. (1986) Mechanics of toric soft lens stabilisation. *Transactions of the British Contact Lens Association Annual Clinical Conference*, **3**, 44–47
3. Westerhout, D. (1989) Toric contact lens fitting. In *Contact Lenses*, A.J. Phillips and J. Stone (eds), Butterworths, London, pp. 505–554
4. Holden, B.A. and Frauenfelder, G. (1975) Principles and practice of correcting astigmatism with soft contact lenses. *Australian Journal of Optometry*, **58**, 279–299

Chapter 23

Presbyopes and bifocal lenses

23.1 Patient selection

23.1.1 New patients

INDICATIONS

- Patients who fulfil the normal criteria for successful contact lens wear.
- Fairly tolerant patients who can accept some compromize in their distance and near vision.
- Patients without exacting visual requirements.

CONTRAINDICATIONS

- Near emmetropes for distance.
- Where there are basic contraindications to contact lens wear.
- Very critical patients.
- Patients who need good sustained close vision for work require particular care.
- Where the reason for fitting is obviously a spectacle dispensing problem.
- Poor handling.

Practical advice

To give prior assessment of adaptation, fit single vision distance first or try disposables if:

- The patient is uncertain about contact lenses.
- There are practitioner doubts about suitability.
- Handling may be a problem.

23.1.2 Existing lens wearers

- Early presbyopes often cope with +0.50D added to the distance correction, usually in one eye.
- Many patients are happy to wear reading spectacles over their contact lenses to avoid both complications and expense.
- Some patients accidentally using monovision because of refractive change are less happy when refitted with bifocals.
- If the patient is a successful hard lens wearer, soft bifocals should not be fitted.

INDICATIONS

- Long-term wearers who do not wish to resume spectacles even for reading.
- Physical problems with spectacles.
- Nuisance value of spectacles for one specific task.

CONTRAINDICATIONS

- Poor volume or quality of tears, common with presbyopes.
- Where tolerance is becoming marginal with single vision lenses.
- Patients taking systemic drugs (e.g. for arthritis or hormone replacement therapy).

23.2 Monovision

Monovision is a technique for correcting presbyopia in which reading power is incorporated into a single-vision contact lens worn usually on the non-dominant eye.

23.2.1 Advantages and disadvantages of monovision

ADVANTAGES

- The least complicated method of dealing with presbyopia.
- It is unnecessary to make any compromise in the fitting.
- Patient acceptability is high, provided that the concept has been explained.

- Stability of vision.
- Patients usually decide rapidly that they can or cannot accept the technique.
- Significantly less expensive than bifocals.

DISADVANTAGES

- Reduced stereopsis, although this is negligible for infinity and peripheral fusion is maintained.
- Some loss of contrast, although this is true of most bifocal lenses.
- Unacceptable blurring may reduce tolerance.
- Cannot be used with monocular patients.
- Requires fairly strong eye dominance.
- Care is required with driving.

23.2.2 Fitting for monovision

- Lenses, hard or soft, are fitted according to normal criteria.
- The non-dominant eye is used for near.
- The left is more often the non-dominant eye; in the UK, this is more practicable for driving.
- The least minus or most plus is found for distance in the dominant eye.
- The minimum plus power for adequate near vision is included for the non-dominant eye.

Practical advice

- If right and left eyes are similar in prescription, the patient can experiment with which eye to use for near.
- If near vision is the main use, try changing the dominance and adapting the method to the patient's needs.
- For occasional optimum distance vision (e.g. prolonged driving), consider prescribing either a third distance lens for the non-dominant eye or spectacles to wear over the lenses.

Partial monovision

A low add of only +0.50 D or +0.75 D often gives sufficient convenience for intermittent near vision (e.g. price tags, menus, headlines) and patients are then happy to use reading spectacles for serious close work.

23.3 Bifocal lens designs

23.3.1 Alternating designs (translating bifocals)

Alternating lenses contain two distinct sectors. These may be either fused or solid portions, or extend across the entire width of the lens (Figure 23.1a,b). Segment lenses are more common, but the concept is equally valid with concentric designs. Distance and near portions can never be used in the same direction of gaze or at the same time. Lens stability and position are controlled by either prism or truncation.

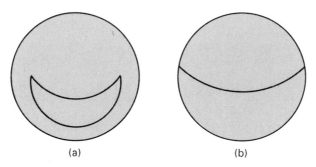

(a)   (b)

Figure 23.1 Bifocal lens design: (a) fused or solid portion; (b) solid portion extending across lens width

FACTORS FOR SUCCESSFUL FITTING

- The lens must move upwards on downward gaze to bring the near portion in front of the pupil area.
- A relatively taut lower lid is necessary; if it is too slack, the lens edge slides across the lower limbus.
- The bottom lid should be no lower than the inferior limbus in order to support the lens.
- There should be minimal disturbance of the lens on blinking or the reading portion is drawn in front of the pupil for distance and the patient complains of variable vision.

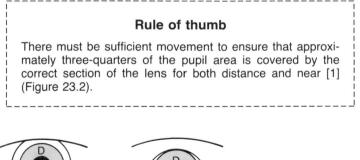

Rule of thumb

There must be sufficient movement to ensure that approximately three-quarters of the pupil area is covered by the correct section of the lens for both distance and near [1] (Figure 23.2).

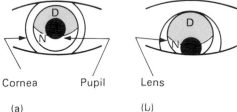

Cornea   Pupil   Lens

(a)   (b)

Figure 23.2 Bifocal lens movement: (a) primary gaze; (b) down gaze (D, distance portion; N, near portion)

23.3.2 Simultaneous designs (non-translating bifocals)

Simultaneous designs essentially provide distance and near vision together and do not rely on lens movement. They are commonly found with concentric or aspheric lenses where they are usually referred to as centre near (CN) and centre distance (CD), or with diffractive designs.

FACTORS FOR SUCCESSFUL FITTING

Stability of fit and the ability to discern between distance and near are important factors. Pupil size is also very significant in the performance of all simultaneous bifocals except diffractive lenses.

One of the main problems with simultaneous bifocals is a loss of contrast sensitivity of the superimposed retinal images. The problem is worse in low illumination and can give particular difficulties at near.

Centre near lenses

- Low illumination with CN concentric types favours distance vision because of the increase in pupil size.

- High illumination with CN concentric types favours near vision because of the decrease in pupil size; thus drivers should wear sunglasses.

- With CN aspherics, the larger the pupil the better the distance vision. Older patients with small pupils may not achieve good distance acuity.

Centre distance lenses

- Low illumination with CD concentric types favours near vision.

- High illumination with CD concentric types favours distance vision; thus sunglasses should be worn to read on a beach.

- With CD aspherics, small pupils make available less reading addition; thus, the older the patient the less suitable for near.

23.4 Fitting PMMA and hard bifocals

23.4.1 Alternating types

FUSED OR SOLID SEGMENTED BIFOCALS

PMMA lenses are ordered with fused segments of different refractive index, whereas hard lenses currently use solid segments with the same refractive index. Fitting is based on the largest feasible TD to permit a typical upcurve segment width of 6 mm.

Distance powers and near addition are determined by refraction. The pupil diameter in average illumination and the distance from the bottom edge of the pupil to the lower lid are measured. The top of the segment is ideally placed one-quarter of the pupil diameter above the pupil margin to enable the

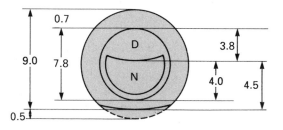

Figure 23.3 Bifocal lens drawn with measurements for ordering (D, distance portion; N, near portion) (After Stone [2])

distance portion to cover approximately three-quarters of the pupil area. Plus lenses require $1.5^\triangle$, minus lenses $2^\triangle$ or more and an allowance is made for the 0.50 mm truncation where this is used. The lens can be drawn with measurements when ordering [2] (Figure 23.3).

Typical specification

C3 7.80:7.80/8.70:8.60/10.50:$\underline{9.50}$ −2.00   Add +2.50
                              9.00

Seg. height 4.50 mm; prism ballast $1.50^\triangle$; truncation 0.50 mm; flat edge

---

Practical advice

- Err on the high side for the segment top, as this can subsequently be modified.
- Increase the truncation if the segment is located too high.
- Solid segment bifocals can cause problems with image jump and diplopia.
- Hard bifocals work best with plus or low minus cases.
- Fused PMMA segments usually fluoresce with UV, so that assessing the segment position is straightforward with a Burton lamp or on the slit lamp.
- Observe the position of solid segments with an ophthalmoscope because they do not fluoresce.

ONE-PIECE HARD BIFOCAL (e.g. TANGENT STREAKS[TM])

Consists of two wide segments meeting at a straight horizontal junction (Figure 23.4), similar to an Executive-type spectacle bifocal.

A trial set is necessary to assess movement of the lens and position of the segment line. A flat fitting is required so that the lens rides onto the lower lid between blinks. A low position is necessary to ensure sufficient clearance between the top of the lens and superior limbus for adequate translation, which is helped by truncation combined with $2^\triangle$. The range of BOZRs is 7.42 mm (45.50 D) to 8.23 mm (41.00 D) and the initial lens is selected on the basis of Table 23.1.

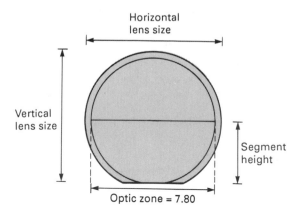

Figure 23.4 Design of Tangent Streak™ one-piece hard bifocal

Table 23.1 Tangent Streak

Corneal astigmatism (D)	Trial lens (BOZR)
0.00 D	'K' + 0.20 mm
0.50 D	'K' + 0.10 mm
>1.00 D	1/4 between flattest and steepest 'K'

The BOZD is a constant 7.80 mm, although there are two standard TDs of 9.90/9.40 mm and 9.40/9.00 mm. The position of the segment is observed with the ophthalmoscope or slit lamp. It is ideally 1.50 mm below the centre of the pupil in distance gaze. In downward gaze, the lens should translate for the segment line to rise slightly above the pupil centre. If the lens is not pushed up by the bottom lid, then more prism or a flatter BOZR should be used. Where the lower lid is below the limbus, a lens should be used with larger TD, less truncation, and higher segment. Example:

HVID: 12.00 mm   Pupil size 4.00 mm   'K' 7.80 × 7.65
BOZR: 7.90 mm; TD 9.90/9.40; seg. height 5.20 mm

Practical advice

- Always use a trial set and take advantage of loan lenses where available.
- Use trial lenses as near as possible to the anticipated BVP

because lenses of different power behave differently on the eye.

- Err on the flat side for the initial trial lens.
- The larger TD is used more frequently.
- If the fluorescein pattern is irregular and difficult to interpret, judge the fit according to movement and translation.
- Lenses are supplied dry and require hydration for 24 h before dispensing.

23.4.2 Simultaneous types

CONCENTRIC BIFOCALS

Concentric bifocals are especially suitable when good near vision is required above eye level, although some patients find the superimposed images difficult to ignore. The diameter of the distance portion is dependent on the pupil size and the lenses must be fitted to centre well with minimum movement. Back or front surface designs are possible (Figure 23.5a,b), although the latter are more frequently fitted [1].

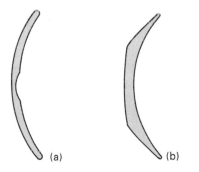

(a)   (b)

Figure 23.5 Concentric bifocals: (a) back surface design; (b) front surface design (from Phillips and Stone, *Contact Lenses*, 3rd edn, Butterworth-Heinemann, by permission)

Front surface

These are CD lenses made as lenticulars, with a central flatter curve giving a small optic area for distance surrounded by a steeper carrier, the radius of which is selected to give the correct power for near. The distance portion varies between 3.00 mm and 5.00 mm and should cover 50% of the pupil area. 4.00 mm is needed in 70% of cases. It is often useful to bias one eye for distance with a larger segment and the other for near with a smaller central area. A stable fit is achieved with large TDs between 9.60 mm and 9.90 mm, although some vertical movement is essential for satisfactory near vision. A low-riding lens works better than a high-riding one.

Typical specification

R and L: 7.80:7.50/8.40:8.60/10.50:9.80 −3.00 Add +2.00
Right seg. size 4.30 mm; Left seg. size 3.50 mm

Practical advice

The lenticular design means that it is possible to:

- Add negative power to the distance area.
- Add positive power to the near carrier.
- Increase to a small extent the size of the distance area.

Back surface

The de Carle lens is a CD design [3] with a very steep central back curve which relies on the partial neutralization effect of the tears. It has a typical radius of about 6.90 mm for an add of +2.50 D and a diameter between 2.00 mm and 4.00 mm. The surrounding annulus for near is used as a bearing surface (*see* Figure 23.5a).

ASPHERIC (e.g. APA)

The APA [4] consists of a paraboloid back surface progressively flattening from apex to periphery. The eccentricity gives a significant increase in plus power away from the apex. The chord diameter of the apical radius is only 0.06 mm, so that flattening occurs over the majority of the lens.

BOZRs range from 6.70 mm to 7.20 mm to allow the lens to be fitted 0.8–1.00 mm steeper than 'K'. This gives apical clearance with uniform bearing on the peripheral cornea.

The TD varies with BOZR from 8.80 mm to 9.60 mm. The optimum fit is the smallest lens which gives centration and stability on blinking, with a preference for fitting steeper with minimum displacement. Centration is important because a decentred lens requires more minus power which neutralizes the plus available for near. A steeper lens adds plus power, so that a change in BOZR can be used to achieve optimum vision.

DIFFRACTIVE BIFOCALS (e.g. DIFFRAX)

Diffractive bifocals consist of a circular phase plate incorporated into the optic zone. The light is made to interfere constructively at two focal points and destructively at other points on the optic axis [5]. The reading addition depends upon the number of rings in the holographic phase plate – the more rings, the higher the add (Figure 23.6). A trial set is essential for fitting, although the design is pupil independent.

Diffrax lenses are made in Polycon II material and have a six-curve construction with a standard TD of 9.50 mm. They are fitted 0.10 mm steeper than 'K' to ensure corneal clearance by the posterior surface and provide good centration to cover the

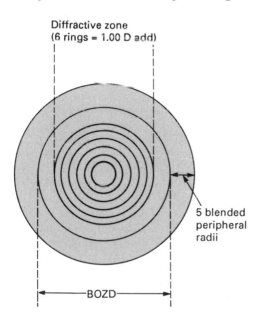

Figure 23.6 Diffractive bifocal (Diffrax design)

pupil area. Distance and near powers are assessed separately and binocular refraction is advisable. There is better differentiation between distance and near vision with adds higher than +1.50 D. The main problems with distance are flare in bright sunshine and lights at night. A '3-D' ghosting effect is sometimes observed at near.

Typical specification

7.60:9.50   +2.00   Add +2.00

23.5 Fitting soft bifocals

23.5.1 Alternating type

Alternating bifocals have not generally proved successful with soft lenses because of the difficulty of large lenses translating effectively. Lenses which have been produced consist of:

● Crescent segments stabilized by truncation and prism ballast.

● Concentric designs with a high minus edge to interact with the lower lid and translate.

23.5.2 Simultaneous types

CONCENTRIC BIFOCALS (SPHERICAL)

Both CD and CN designs are available. The decision should be made whether distance or near is more important and a lens fitted with that particular requirement in the centre (e.g. VDU operators are more likely to need a CN design and drivers a CD design). Lenses are pupil dependent, so that a trial set is necessary for both fitting and power determination. The size of the central portion, whether distance or near, determines the visual bias and potential success of the lens.

The optimum fitting should give minimal movement with good centration. The initial lens, however, should be the flattest reasonable choice because older, presbyopic eyes have a reduced volume of tears and less free lens movement over the conjunctiva.

The position of the central portion within the pupil area is more easily checked with either the retinoscope or ophthalmoscope than with the slit lamp. A decentred segment is unlikely to give good vision. It is often advantageous to use different segment sizes in each eye, biasing one towards distance and the other towards near.

Centre near (e.g. Alges)

The Alges lens has a TD of 14.00 mm and radii of 8.90 mm and 8.60 mm. The diameters used for the central near portion are 2.35 mm, 2.55 mm and less often 2.12 mm. There are four adds from +2.00 D to +3.50 D in 0.50 D steps, and approximately 1.00 D more plus is required for near compared with spectacles. The lens design is very thin so that handling can be difficult.

Typical specification

R. and L. 8.60:14.00   −3.00   Add +2.50
Right seg. 2.35 mm; Left seg. 2.55 mm

Centre distance (e.g. Ciba Bisoft)

The Bisoft design has 'steep' and 'flat' fittings with TDs of 13.00 mm and 13.80 mm. Distance powers range from −10.00 D to +7.00, with adds from +1.50 D to +4.00 D, both in 0.25 D steps. The diameters of the central distance portion are either 3.2 mm or 3.8 mm.

ASPHERIC BIFOCALS

Back surface aspheric (e.g. Hydrocurve II)

A CD design with progressively increasing near addition towards a maximum of +1.50 at the periphery. It is a 'one-fit' lens in a 45% water content material selected entirely on the basis of distance vision. The power range is from −6.00 D to + 4.00 D. Optimum performance is achieved with good centration under conditions of average illumination and pupil size. The lens works better for early presbyopes because of the limited reading add and can be made more successful with over-plus in one or both eyes if fitted in combination with another type.

Typical specification

9.00:14.80   −3.00

Front surface aspheric (e.g. Nissel PS45)

A CN design based on the over-correction of spherical aberration. The constant near power of +2.00 D becomes increasingly less positive towards the periphery. Distance vision is better with large pupils, whereas near is relatively unaffected by pupil size. Distance powers range from +4.00 D to −6.00 D and although it is a 'one-fit' design, good centration is essential. A full trial set is necessary to assess vision by means of lenses within 0.50 D of the anticipated result using binocular refraction. Lenses are essentially fitted for near vision, often with under-correction in the dominant eye and over-plus in the other. Examples:

Spectacle Rx	Initial trial lens
−2.00 D	plano
+3.00 D	+5.00 D

DIFFRACTIVE BIFOCALS (e.g. ECHELON)

The optical principle is similar to that of the hard Diffrax bifocal and is based on Fresnel-type diffraction facets (Echelettes) less than 3 μm in depth. Chromatic aberration is reduced and there is virtually no pupil dependence. With distance vision, however, light scatter is observed around point sources and some patients have problems with sunlight and driving at night. At near, there is sometimes a ghosting or '3-D' effect.

The lens is a 'one-fit' design in 38% HEMA. Distance powers range from +4.00 D to −6.00 D, with near adds of +1.50 D and +2.00 D.

Typical specification

8.70:13.80   −3.00   Add +2.00

COMBINATIONS

A combination of one single vision lens and one bifocal, or two different designs of bifocal, increases the chance of success. The following combinations can be tried to give better distance vision to a dominant right eye:

Right eye	*Left eye*
Distance single vision	Centre near bifocal
Centre distance bifocal	Centre near bifocal
Centre distance bifocal	Near single vision

General advice

- Have available a variety of soft bifocals in order to fit the majority of suitable patients.

- It is essential to use trial lenses to obtain any idea of potential success for any particular type of bifocal.

- Try different combinations of bifocals and single vision lenses according to eye dominance.

- Avoid fitting poor lens handlers because of the potential expense with breakages.

- Monovision has a higher success rate than bifocals.

- Do not fit patients with very small pupils of 3 mm or less. They are unable to use the area beyond the central power.

References

1. de Carle, J.T. (1989) Bifocal and multifocal contact lenses. In *Contact Lenses*, A.J. Phillips and J. Stone (eds), Butterworths, London, pp. 595–624
2. Stone, J. (1983) Fitting bifocal contact lenses. *Ophthalmic Optician*, **23**, 350–352
3. de Carle, J.T. (1959) The de Carle bifocal contact lens. *Contacto*, **3**, 5–9
4. Goldberg, J.B. and Lowther, G.E. (1986) The variable near powers of aspheric multifocal corneal lenses: a review. *International Eyecare*, **2**, 265–270
5. Freeman, M.H. and Stone, J. (1987) A new diffractive bifocal contact lens. *Transactions of the British Contact Lens Association Annual Clinical Conference*, **4**, 15–22

Chapter 24

Special lens features and applications

24.1 Lens identification

24.1.1 Hard and PMMA lenses

- A single dot engraved on the right lens is the British Standards recommendation.
- 'R' and 'L' engravings. Sometimes only the 'R' is used.
- Partial or complete lens specification is engraved by some manufacturers (e.g. Ciba). This is intended for practitioner rather than patient information.
- Location of cylinder axis or prism base.
- Position of segment to assist bifocal fitting.
- Aphakics and hypermetropes, with poor unaided near vision, sometimes find it useful to have right and left lenses made in different tints.
- A black dot is easier to see on high negative lenses than an engraving.

24.1.2 Soft lenses

Modern laser techniques have largely eliminated earlier problems with mechanical engravings which could either develop fractures or attract deposits. Information can also be imprinted onto the lens photographically and the same method can be used by the practitioner to mark 'R' and 'L'.

- 'R' and 'L' engravings.
- 'R' and 'L' photographic markings.
- A code, serial or lot number.
- Details of partial or complete lens specification.
- Location of cylinder axis or prism base.
- Position of segment to assist bifocal fitting.

24.2 Tinted, cosmetic and prosthetic lenses

Lenses are tinted for a variety of reasons:

- To reduce adaptive photophobia.
- To assist handling.
- To enhance or change the natural eye colour.
- To reduce photophobia in albinism and aphakia.
- For identification.
- To improve colour vision (*see* Section 24.2.2).

The potential disadvantages of tinted lenses are:

- Change in colour values.
- Difficulty with night vision, particularly driving.
- Possible toxicity of dyes.

Cosmetic lenses, in this context, may be defined as those used to change the colour of the eyes, whereas prosthetic lenses are used to conceal unsightly scarring or abnormalities of the iris.

24.2.1 Hard lenses

Most modern hard lenses are available in a fairly restricted range of tints. Many materials are made only in pale blue and do not give the option of clear lenses. Grey (and sometimes brown) is usually possibly. Green is not available in several widely used materials, and in addition the colour reproducibility tends to be unreliable. There is generally poor consistency of colour between different batches of most tints and patients should be advised of the potential problem with replacement lenses.

Hand-painted cosmetic and prosthetic lenses are limited to stable, relatively low *Dk* materials such as XL20 (Nissel).

24.2.2 PMMA lenses

PMMA lenses, in contrast, are available in a wide range of stable, consistently reproducible tints. The most common, standardly used colours are marked with an asterisk.

Grey		Brown	
911	very pale grey	2285-1*	light brown
912*	light grey (the most common)	2285-2	medium brown
512	medium grey/brown	2285	dark brown
999	dark grey		

Blue		*Green*	
1077-1*	light blue	2240-2*	light green
700	light/medium blue/violet	2240-3	medium green
1077-3	medium blue	600	bright green
1077-2	dark blue	2240-1	dark green

Other tints

Yellow	200
Amber	300
Red	2241-1, 400
Pink	2241-2
Lavender	2242-2
Violet	10910

Clinical quality (CQ) materials use inert carbon particles within the monomer to avoid any possiᵘle ᵗoxic effect of dyes in commercial grade PMMA:

Clear
Very light grey/brown– 9042 (previously 911 CQ)
Light grey/brown   – 9043 (previously 912 CQ)

COSMETIC AND PROSTHETIC LENSES

Cosmetic and prosthetic corneal lenses are available with painted laminated inserts (e.g. Nissel). These are colour matched from photographs or sets of sample iris buttons and are usually painted by hand with the appropriate clear or black pupil. Although they give excellent cosmetic results, there are several difficulties associated with the use of corrective lenses:

● They are necessarily thick with large total diameters (about 11.50 mm) to give good corneal coverage and appearance.

● Comfort is often poor with limited wearing time.

● There is a high risk of corneal oedema.

● The artificial pupils often give visual disturbance on blinking.

● There is a tunnel vision effect, with restricted field of view.

● It is not possible to assess the fitting of opaque lenses with fluorescein.

Some of these problems are overcome with the use of scleral lenses (*see* Section 31.1).

THE X-CHROM LENS

A specialized application of tinting is the monocular use of the dark red X-chrom lens. Its particular transmission characteristics are reported to enhance colour discrimination in patients with red–green deficiency [1].

24.2.3 Soft lenses

There is much less clinical need for tinted soft lenses because of the low incidence of adaptive photophobia. Numerous laboratories, however, offer a range of tints for mainly cosmetic reasons. Opaque and semi-opaque lenses are also available for cosmetic and prosthetic fitting. The most common variations are shown in Figure 24.1(a–d).

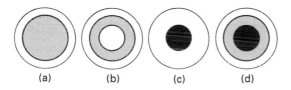

(a)   (b)   (c)   (d)

Figure 24.1 Variations possible with soft lens tints: (a) tinted iris with clear peripheral annulus; (b) tinted iris with clear peripheral annulus and clear pupil; (c) black (opaque) pupil on clear lens; (d) tinted iris with clear peripheral annulus and black (opaque) pupil.

(a) Tinted iris with clear peripheral annulus. The iris diameter is usually standardized at 11.30 mm, with a clear periphery to give a natural appearance on the eye. Some laboratories offer both a range of tints and colour densities. Very pale, handling tints are also possible (e.g. Optima, Ciba soft, Omniflex).
(b) Tinted iris with clear pupil and clear peripheral annulus. The clear pupil partially avoids problems with changed colour values and light reduction at night. The cosmetic appearance is not as satisfactory for many patients as a completely tinted iris.
(c) Clear lens with black pupil. Used for occlusion or prosthetic reasons.
(d) Tinted iris with black pupil and clear peripheral annulus. Used for occlusion or prosthetic reasons.

Soft lenses are also produced with inhibitors, specifically to eliminate the ultraviolet part of the spectrum (e.g. Permaflex) and 'sun filters' (e.g. Lunelle).

OPAQUE PAINTED AND PRINTED LENSES

For both cosmetic and prosthetic purposes it is also possible to manufacture soft lenses with an opaque laminated backing or insert. This may be either painted or printed with clear or black pupils. Depending upon the laboratory, a limitless range of colours and cosmetic effects is possible, but the additional lens thickness of inserts can cause problems with comfort and oedema. Despite their greater stability on the eye compared with hard lenses, opaque corrective soft lenses with a clear pupil can also give visual disturbance on blinking and a reduced field of view.

DOT MATRIX LENSES

Another successful cosmetic approach is the manufacture of lenses with coloured dot matrix patterns (e.g. Wesley/Jessen, Durasoft; Pilkington, Mystique). These avoid the visual problems which occur with opaque lenses. A further refinement of design to overcome the restricted field of view is to have the patterns more widely spaced towards the pupil area (e.g. Durasoft).

General advice

- Order most hard and PMMA lenses with a light tint to assist handling and reduce adaptive photophobia.
- Do not fit tinted soft lenses just for the sake of it. Unless a specific cosmetic effect is required or the lens type is made with a standard handling tint, the advantages are outweighed by practical difficulties of colour matching, time delays, colour fading and the constraints of which solution systems can be used.
- Avoid tints where colour values are important (e.g. artists).
- Care is required with the choice of solutions for tinted and cosmetic soft lenses. Oxidizing systems, especially those based on chlorine, can cause colour fading or laminates to peel apart.
- It is difficult to persuade many patients, particularly emmetropes, that tinted and cosmetic lenses are more than just a fashion accessory. Careful explanation is necessary that they must be fitted with the same skill and

accuracy as conventional lenses and that proper care and maintenance are essential to avoid the risk of infection.

- The effect of a tinted lens cannot be judged unless placed on the eye. The final result is a combination of lens tint, iris colour and ambient lighting.
- To enhance eye colour do not use a tint which is too dark. The most pleasing cosmetic effect is usually achieved with a subtle colour change.
- Dark brown eyes are virtually unaffected by purely tinted lenses. Use opaque or dot matrix soft lenses to give a cosmetic colour change.
- Grey eyes respond well to blue and green tints.
- Light and medium brown eyes may sometimes respond to green tints.
- Brown eyes can sometimes be lightened with a yellow tint.
- Blue eyes may become brown with an orange tint.

24.3 Fenestration

USES OF FENESTRATION

PMMA (and occasionally modern hard) lenses are ventilated to:

- Resolve corneal oedema.
- Improve comfort in hot stuffy atmospheres.
- Lengthen wearing time.
- Reduce the risk of overwear syndrome (see Section 28.1).
- Improve tear flow beneath the lens.
- Reduce spectacle blur.
- Give faster adaptation.
- Improve frothing and dimpling.
- Prevent adhesion.

PROBLEMS WITH FENESTRATION

- Discomfort in some cases.
- Visual disturbance on blinking with about 20% of patients.
- Lenses are weakened mechanically with the risk of cracking.
- The holes can become blocked with secretions from the tears.

Practical advice

- Use single holes for lenses smaller than 9.00 mm; two or more for larger total diameters.
- The size is usually 0.25–0.4 mm, but can vary from 0.1 mm to as large as 1 mm.
- Position fenestrations 1–2 mm off centre with a minus lens to reduce the risk of cracking and allow the holes to cover a greater area of the cornea as the lens rotates on blinking.
- Avoid placing a peripheral hole on a transitional bearing area.
- If there is some doubt as to how the patient will react to the fenestrations, modify one lens at a time.
- Err slightly on the small side, as the ventilation holes can subsequently be enlarged.
- Instruct the patient to maintain the patency of the holes with the careful use of a soft, boxwood cocktail stick.
- Despite the obvious, always instruct the laboratory 'countersunk and very well polished'.

24.4 Overseas prescriptions

Most soft lens specifications are international. Some differences may be found with hard and PMMA lenses. Prescriptions from continental Europe may be written in the order of radius (R_o), power (D), diameter ($\emptyset$). Example: 7.80 −3.00 9.40

US prescriptions often give the BOZR (base curve or BCR) derived from keratometry fitting in dioptres. This is converted to millimetres using $n = 1.3375$. Peripheral (intermediate or secondary) curves are usually followed by their width and the overall diameter (OAD) in millimetres. The final back peripheral curve is usually called a 'bevel'. A convex, front peripheral curve to reduce the edge thickness of minus lenses is sometimes called a 'CN bevel'. Example:

BCR   45.00 D   OZ 7.80 mm   OAD 9.60 mm
SCR   39.25 D   (0.6 mm)
Bevel 32.12 D   (0.3 mm)

is equivalent to 7.50:7.80/8.60:9.00/10.50:9.60.

24.5 Contact lenses and sport

24.5.1 Advantages and disadvantages

Contact lenses offer considerable advantages over spectacles for sport.

ADVANTAGES

- Larger field of view.
- Unaffected by bad weather.
- With contact sports, both player and opponents are safer with no spectacle frame.

DISADVANTAGES

Disadvantages relate mainly to hard lenses:

- Loss or displacement.
- Increased photophobia.
- Foreign bodies.

Because of these potential disadvantages, the governing bodies of certain sports may disallow the use of certain types of contact lens (e.g. rally driving, horse-racing).

24.5.2 Lens types

Soft lenses

Stability is the prime consideration with sport. The lens must give virtually no risk of loss from the eye, even with contact sports; must avoid the intrusion of foreign bodies; and must give consistent vision despite rapid eye movements. Soft lenses are therefore the first choice in most cases. For serious sporting use where optimum acuity is required (e.g. cricket), toric soft lenses are often preferable to hard, even to correct quite small degrees of astigmatism.

The main disadvantage is lens dehydration (*see* Section 17.3).

Hard lenses

For less serious sport, hard lens wearers may well find that they can continue with existing lenses. Hard lenses can also be fitted deliberately larger and tighter than PMMA. They are specifically indicated where optimum acuity is required (e.g. pistol-shooting), and in the case of flying the authorities may insist on their use to the exclusion of soft.

Scleral lenses

Scleral lenses (see Chapter 14) give maximum stability of vision with no risk of loss. Their disadvantages are difficulty of fitting and limited wearing time. They are therefore used only rarely, but have occasional application for aquatic sports such as water polo or canoeing where the head may be under water for a relatively long period.

24.5.3 Specific applications

Swimming

Hard lenses, unless large and tight with a small palpebral aperture, are usually contraindicated because of the high risk of loss. Soft lenses, if used carefully, have been worn fairly successfully. Some patients are very sensitive to chlorine absorbed by the lenses and may show conjunctival injection for several hours after exposure. This can even occur when lenses have been removed during swimming, but replaced before the chlorine has been eliminated from the eyes.

Another factor is the saline concentration of sea water, since soft lenses fit more loosely in hypertonic solution. This could be used to advantage by rinsing lenses with hypotonic solution to tighten the fitting prior to swimming.

It should also be remembered that swimming pools are a frequent source of ocular infection, and micro-organisms such as *Acanthamoeba* may be unaffected by chlorine disinfection.

Diving

Good results have been obtained with various water content soft lenses when used for scuba-diving, with little risk of displacement. Air bubbles tend to form beneath lenses at depths of about 150 ft (45 m), but less with soft than hard which are generally contraindicated for this reason [2].

Water replacing air in front of the cornea reduces its refracting power by about 40.00 D. Scleral lenses have therefore been designed either with a flat-fronted air cell or with a high index glass anterior surface [3].

Skiing

Most forms of contact lens prove very successful for skiing. It is essential to use either goggles or large sunglasses to give protection from wind and cold and prevent soft lens dehydration.

Climbing at high altitude

High *Dk* hard or high water content soft lenses should be used because of the reduced level of oxygen in the atmosphere at high altitude [4]. Extended wear may well be preferred to avoid cold weather difficulties with both handling and solutions.

Shooting

Competition shooting usually requires the precision and stability of hard lens acuity. The binocular balance is important. Depending upon the type of weapon, it is sometimes necessary either to fog the alternate eye or under-correct the fixating eye to assist focusing on the front sight.

References

1. Zeltzer, H. (1982) *X-Chrom Manual*, 2nd edn, The X-Chrom Corp., Waltham, USA
2. Molinari, J. and Socks, J. (1987) Effect of hyperbaric conditions on corneal physiology with hydrogel lenses. *Journal of the British Contact Lens Association* (Scientific Meetings 1987), p. 17
3. Douthwaite, W.A. (1987) *Contact Lens Optics*, Butterworths, London
4. Clarke, C. (1976) Contact lenses at high altitude *British Journal of Ophthalmology*, 60, 170 180

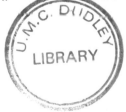

Chapter 25

Care systems

25.1 Components of solutions

All contact lens solutions are produced according to 'general principles of formulation' and 'good manufacturing practice'.

BUFFERS

Buffers (e.g. sodium phosphate, borate or bicarbonate) are included where there is a need to keep the pH within the narrow limits necessary for contact lens wear (pH 6–8).

PRESERVATIVES

Preservatives restrict the growth of micro-organisms and maintain the sterility of the solution remaining in the bottle and in the contact lens case. Typical examples are given below.

Benzalkonium chloride (BAK)

Frequently used with PMMA lenses. It destabilizes the tear film in concentrations over 0.004%, so wetting solutions or rewetting drops do not exceed this concentration. The majority of soaking and cleaning solutions can use 0.004–0.01% because they do not come into contact with the eye. Its use with modern hard lenses has been questioned because of surface adsorption [1].
Benzalkonium chloride is never used with soft lenses because of its toxicity to the cornea in large or sustained doses.

Chlorhexidine digluconate (CHX)

Usually included with other preservative systems in a concentration of 0.006% for hard lens solutions. If it is used alone, the kill time is slow and lenses must be stored for a minimum of

10 h. Soft lens solutions employ a reduced concentration of 0.002–0.005% (e.g. Bausch and Lomb Wetting and Soaking).

Thiomersal

A mercurial derivative used in concentrations of 0.001–0.002% with both hard and soft lens solutions, more often found with the latter. Thiomersal is effective against fungi, but toxic reactions are fairly common. It is slow acting as a preservative and so is usually incorporated with chlorhexidine or EDTA (e.g. Hydrosoak).

Phenylmercuric nitrate

Found in some multi-purpose hard lens solutions in a concentration of 0.004% (e.g. Clean-N-Soak).

Chlorbutol

Binds to CAB and now uncommon due to its volatile nature. Used in concentrations of 0.4% (e.g. Sterisoak, Liquifilm Tears).

Quaternary ammonias

Used in soft lens soaking solutions in concentrations of 0.013–0.03% (e.g. Hydrocare Cleaning and Soaking).

Sorbic acid

Used in surfactant cleaners with a concentration of 0.1% (e.g. Pliagel).

TONICITY AGENTS (invariably SODIUM CHLORIDE)

To adjust the salt concentration and ensure compatibility with the tears.

VISCOSITY AGENTS (e.g. METHYL CELLULOSE)

To improve the wetting time and comfort of the solution.

WETTING AGENTS (e.g. POLYVINYL ALCOHOL, POLYSORBATE 80)

To help the solution spread across the lens surface. Also found in soft lens disinfection solutions (e.g. polyvinyl pyrrolidone).

CHELATING AGENTS (e.g. ETHYLENEDIAMINE TETRAACETIC ACID (EDTA) KNOWN AS SODIUM EDETATE)

Found in concentrations of 0.01–0.2%. Used to enhance the action of preservatives, especially benzalkonium chloride with which it has a synergistic action. The main exceptions are mercurial derivatives.

25.2 Solutions for hard and PMMA lenses

Compared with PMMA, hard lens surfaces are more prone to deposits and interaction with some formulations.

25.2.1 Wetting solutions

Wetting solutions are used on insertion to act as a cushion between the lens and cornea. They also enhance the spread of tears across the lens surface, although the effect only lasts for a maximum of 15 min and sometimes for as little as 5 s [2].

Formulation: tonicity agent; viscosity agent; wetting agent; preservatives; chelating agent.

25.2.2 Soaking solutions

Soaking solutions keep lenses hydrated during overnight storage in a sterile bacteriocidal environment. They facilitate good surface wetting and assist the removal of deposits. Hydration is important to maintain the correct BOZR both for modern hard lens materials [3] and for PMMA over about −10.00 D [4].

Formulation: tonicity agent; wetting agent; detergent; preservatives; chelating agent.

25.2.3 Cleaning solutions

Cleaning solutions remove surface debris such as lipids and mucus and enhance the disinfecting action of the soaking solution. They help keep the lens clean during wear and give a light surface polishing effect if they contain particles in suspension.

Formulation: detergent; preservatives; chelating agent.

Practical advice

- Take care not to cause an inadvertent power change with the polishing action.
- Take care with cleaners containing only an organic solvent (e.g. isopropyl alcohol) to avoid upsetting the surface wetting properties of some hard lens materials, especially fluoropolymers [5].

25.2.4 Multi-purpose solutions

These combine all of the above functions, but usually with some loss of efficiency:

- Wetting, soaking and cleaning (e.g. Total)
- Soaking and cleaning (e.g. Clean-N-Soak).
- Cleaning and wetting (e.g. Steri-Clens).
- Wetting and soaking (e.g. Bausch and Lomb).

Formulation: wetting agent; detergent; preservatives; chelating agent.

25.2.5 Rewetting solutions (comfort drops)

Comfort drops are used to rewet lenses while they are worn, especially in dry environments.

Formulation: wetting agent; preservatives; chelating agent.

25.2.6 Enzyme tablets

Proteinaceous films require enzyme removal with some hard lens materials, particularly silicone acrylates.

Formulation (see Section 25.4.4).

Practical advice

- Depending upon the active ingredient, patients find it much more convenient to leave lenses soaking overnight.
- Enzymes are often not required with fluoropolymers and rarely with CAB.
- Advise hay fever sufferers to use them more frequently in the spring and early summer.

25.3 Solutions for soft lenses

The general principles for soft lens solutions are similar to those of hard, but there are potentially more difficulties because of the possibility of interaction with the material. Viscosity agents are not generally employed and the pattern of use is often different, since many solutions must be partnered to ensure their complete anti-microbial efficacy.

25.4 Disinfection

Disinfection may be by means of either *chemicals* (cold) or *heat*.

25.4.1 Chemical disinfection

Cold disinfection uses either preserved chemicals or unpreserved oxidative systems.

Preserved soaking solutions

Used for overnight storage (e.g. Prymesoak, Hydrosoak).
Formulation: tonicity agent; wetting agent; preservative; buffer; detergent.

Saline

Normal (0.9%) saline may be either buffered or unbuffered and is available in the following formats:

● Preserved in multi-dose bottles.

● Unpreserved in unit dose form (e.g. Amidose).

● Unpreserved in aerosol form (e.g. Solusal, Lens Plus).

● Drip-feed bags with one-way valve (not obtainable in the UK except in some hospital departments).

N.B. Home-made saline, using purified water, ceased in the UK in 1988 with the withdrawal of salt tablets. *Acanthamoeba* infection in the USA has been linked to home-made saline [6].

Tap water

The OptimEyes tablet, containing 0.004% chlorhexidine, when dissolved in *rising mains water* creates a simple and inexpensive disinfection system.

Tap water alone should not be used for soft lens storage and insertion because of the risk of microbial contamination; trace metals and salts; and lens sticking as a result of hypotonicity. Rising mains water can be used to flush contaminated lenses, but they must be fully disinfected afterwards.

OXIDATIVE SYSTEMS

Oxidative systems are generally unpreserved and use hydrogen peroxide- or chlorine-based compounds as the disinfecting agent.

Hydrogen peroxide (H_2O_2)

Most peroxide systems use a 3% concentration. They include a sodium or phosphate stabilizer to prevent the rapid decompensation of the otherwise unstable H_2O_2 [7].

Cleaners can be included with the peroxide solution. Examples are Consept (a surfactant) and Ultrazyme (an enzyme tablet).

Advantages of hydrogen peroxide

- No reaction to preservatives.
- Efficient method of disinfecting.
- Enhances cleaning.
- A surface or enzyme cleaner can sometimes be avoided.
- Prolongs lens life.
- Less risk of 'red eye' reaction with extended wear.

Disadvantages of hydrogen peroxide

- The peroxide must be neutralized.
- The neutralizing time is sometimes lengthy.
- Complicated to use and understand.
- High water content materials may deteriorate with prolonged storage in peroxide.
- Occasional allergies.
- The peroxide may lose its efficacy if kept too long (e.g. extended wear).
- Bulky for travel.

● Expensive.

● Possibility of patient error.

Three types of neutralization are available:

(1) *Catalytic*. Uses either catalase, a naturally occurring bovine catalyst which is highly specific for the speedy decomposition of hydrogen peroxide (e.g. Oxysept) or a platinum-coated disc (e.g. Septicon or AOSept). The neutralization does not depend on the concentration of the catalyst and no by-products are formed except water and oxygen. The platinum disc is much slower than the catalase because the molecules have to migrate through the buffered saline to the disc surface instead of being evenly distributed throughout the solution. The disc needs replacing every 3 months (sooner with some patients). If the neutralizing solution is buffered to a high pH (e.g. AOSept), the kill time is slower.

(2) *Reactive*. Chemicals such as sodium pyruvate (e.g. 10:10, Mira-Sept) or sodium thiosulphate (Perform) initiate an oxidation–reduction reaction which causes the hydrogen peroxide to decompose. The speed and degree of neutralization depend upon concentration and temperature. By-products are formed such as sodium acetate, carbon dioxide and water (10:10); or sodium tetrathionate and sodium hydroxide (Perform).

(3) *Dilution*. The peroxide is diluted by rinsing and soaking in saline (e.g. Quik-Sept). The efficacy depends on the number of times the procedure is carried out.

Chlorine systems

Chlorine-based systems contain active ingredients such as sodium dichloroisocyanurate (e.g. Softab) or *para*-dichloro-sulphamoyl benzoic acid (e.g. Aerotab).

Advantages of chlorine

● One-step systems which help compliance.

● Neutralization unnecessary.

● Unpreserved saline is the only solution used, either to dissolve the tablet or rinse the lens before use.

● Less irritation with patient error.

● Easy to understand.

- Minimum bulk and good for travel.
- Less expensive than peroxide.
- Useful for disinfecting trial lenses.

Disadvantages of chlorine

- Residual traces of the disinfecting agent may be present on lens insertion.
- Slow kill time so overnight disinfection required.
- An effective surfactant cleaner is essential.
- May be confused with enzyme tablets.
- Patient may forget to add the tablet.
- Lenses have shorter life span than with H_2O_2.
- Ineffective against *Acanthamoeba*.
- Tinted soft lenses may fade.

25.4.2 Heat disinfection

Heat disinfection is generally carried out using unpreserved normal saline at a pasteurization temperature of 70–80°C. The addition of sodium edetate gives calcium-removing properties. Lenses must always be allowed to cool before insertion.

Advantages of heat disinfection

- Easy to use.
- Economical.
- Efficient at killing micro-organisms.
- Suitable for disposable lenses.

Disadvantages of heat disinfection

- Difficult for travel.
- Denatures protein onto the lens surface.
- Accelerates lens ageing.
- Routine surfactant and enzyme cleaning essential.

Methods

- Heating unit, preferably thermostatic and time controlled.

- Vacuum flask or saucepan. The lens case is placed in boiling water for 10 min after which the lenses are allowed to cool.
- Microwave where the kill time is less than 30 s [8].

25.4.3 Cleaning solutions

Formulation: surface-active agents; preservatives.

In addition to cleaners specifically formulated for soft lenses (e.g. Hydron Cleaning), hard lens cleaners which do not contain benzalkonium chloride can be used. A surfactant–polymeric bead cleaner (Polyclens) combines a cleaning agent with microscopic, polystyrene-like beads [9].

Daily surface cleaning is important to:

- Remove lipids, inorganic deposits, some proteins and insoluble contaminants by manual action.
- Overcome the hydrophobicity of oily deposits with surface-active agents.
- Assist chemical disinfection by removing deposits that could interfere with antibacterial activity.
- Remove contaminants that supply nutrients to bacteria.

Other cleaning methods

- Ultrasonic units.
- Ultraviolet units.
- Spinning devices.

25.4.4 Periodic cleaners

ENZYME TABLETS

Enzyme tablets are used for the removal of protein from the lens surface. Weekly cleaning is suggested, but patients on peroxide are able to use them less frequently. Tablets are dissolved in either saline or distilled water.

Formulation: papain (Hydrocare or Bausch and Lomb); subtilisin A (Ultrazyme); pancreatin (Clenzyme); lipase, pronase, protease, sodium edetate (Amiclair).

Practical advice

- Where papain causes an adverse reaction, especially with high water content lenses, reduce the soaking time to 15 min.
- Hydrogen peroxide breaks down residual papain and should be used after the enzyme cleaner.
- Advise hay fever sufferers to use them more frequently in the spring and early summer.

25.4.5 Professional cleaners

Strong oxidizing agents (e.g. Liprofin; Monoclens) are used by the practitioner for intensive cleaning and rejuvenation. Their action is enhanced by means of tonicity changes and should not be used more than once on a lens because of dimensional changes. High water content lenses are more susceptible and should be treated at a lower temperature for a shorter period of time (*see* Section 4.3.1).

Practical advice

A very small number of patients can give an extreme sensitivity reaction to professional cleaners, however thoroughly lenses are rinsed and boiled out in saline after use.

References

1. Hoffman, W.C. (1987) Ending the BAK-RGP controversy. *Optician*, 193(5095), 31–32
2. Doane, M.G. (1988) *In vivo* measurement of contact lens wetting. *Transactions of the British Contact Lens Association Annual Clinical Conference*, 5, 110–111
3. Pearson, R.M. (1977) Dimensional stability of several hard contact lens materials. *American Journal of Optometry and Physiological Optics*, 54, 826–833
4. Phillips, A.J. (1969) Alterations in curvature of the finished corneal lens. *Ophthalmic Optician*, 9, 980–1110
5. Lowther, G.E. (1987) Effect of some solutions on HGP contact lens parameters. *Journal of the American Optometric Association*, 58, 188–192
6. Stehr-Green, J. (1989) The epidemiology of Acanthamoeba keratitis in the United States. *American Journal of Ophthalmology*, 107, 331
7. Gyulai, P., Dziabo, A., Kelly, W., Kiral, R. and Hayes Powell, C. (1988) Relative neutralization ability of six hydrogen peroxide disinfection systems. *Optician*, 195(5134), 25–32

8. Harris, M., Rechberger, J., Grant, T. and Holden, B.A. (1990) In-office microwave disinfection of soft contact lenses. *Optometry and Visual Science*, **67**, 129–132
9. Fowler, S.A. and Allansmith, M.R. (1984) Removal of soft lens deposits with surfactant–polymeric bead cleaner. *Contact Lens Association of Ophthalmologists Journal*, **10**, 229–231

Chapter 26

Lens collection and patient instruction

26.1 Lens collection

Insertion of lenses

The lenses are inserted after verification and given time to settle before assessing acuities and fitting. An existing wearer needs only a few minutes, whereas a new patient requires 10–20 min depending upon lens type.

Assessment of vision

The visual assessment should confirm that acuities are the same as or better than those achieved during initial fitting.

Assessment of fitting

This should confirm:

- That the fitting appears as originally intended.
- That the lenses have been accurately made. Apart from the main parameters, the practitioner should consider other factors such as blending, lenticulation, thickness and edge shape.
- That the fitting appears satisfactory, even if the previous two criteria are met.
- Whether any discomfort is normal or excessive.

26.2 Insertion and removal

Patients often need to realize that handling is a hurdle to overcome, but has little to do with comfort, vision or eventual wearing time. Insertion should always be done over a flat surface or closed sink, while removal can be into the cupped hand for hard lenses. Patients should be taught initially with a mirror, but it is ultimately better to manage without. Soft and hard lens insertion follow the same pattern, but removal is different.

26.2.1 Hard lenses

Insertion

The lens is cleaned, rinsed and wetted. The lids are held firmly apart while the patient looks at the reflection of the eye in a mirror. The head may be either vertical or horizontal and the lens is placed onto the cornea with the first or second finger of the dominant hand.

Practical advice

- The alternate eye must be kept open to prevent Bell's phenomenon.
- The lids should be held from underneath the base of the lashes to prevent reflex blinking.
- Reassure the patient that the lens does no harm on the sclera and cannot get lost 'behind the eye'.
- Show the patient how to recentre the lens with indirect finger pressure on the lid margins or by massaging through the closed lids.

Removal

The eye must be held open wide enough for the taut lids to eject the lens behind by means of blinking and:

- One finger pulling slightly upwards from the outer canthus.
- Two fingers from the same hand pulling from the lid margins.
- Two fingers, one from each hand, pulling with a sideways scissors motion.
- Two fingers, one from each hand, positioned vertically and pushing the lid margins against the globe of the eye and towards each other. This method, although more difficult to learn, is more consistently reliable.

- Holding the lids firmly and turning the eye nasally.

If all of these methods fail, a moistened suction holder can be applied perpendicular to the centre of the lens.

Practical advice

The patient should not be allowed to leave before being competent at lens removal (insertion can be safely practised at home).

26.2.2 Soft lenses

Insertion

The general principles are the same as for hard lenses. The key difference is that as lenses are self-centring patients need not be concerned if they are inserted out of position. Where near fixation is uncontrollable, especially with hypermetropes, lenses can be inserted onto the inferior sclera while looking upwards at a distant fixation target.

Practical advice

- To stop lens ejection at the moment of insertion because of an air bubble, advise the patient to take both hands away and look down slowly. The eyes should be gently closed and the lids squeezed together to remove the bubble.
- A dry finger helps stop the lens reversing.
- Allow ultra-thin lenses to dry on the finger for about 20 s to help insertion.
- With ultra-thins it may be necessary to pull the upper lid over the lens to prevent the lens rolling out of the eye on lid closure.
- If the lens is uncomfortable on insertion, it should be slid onto the temporal sclera and allowed to recentre. This usually dislodges a foreign body, make-up or very small air bubble. The lens should be removed, rinsed and reinserted if discomfort persists.

Removal

Hard lens pulling methods do not generally work with soft lenses. They are removed by:

● Sliding the lens onto the temporal or inferior sclera and pinching out.

● Pinching directly off the cornea (this is a less satisfactory method because of the risk of scratching the cornea).

● Squeezing at the edge of the lens with the upper and lower lid margins to create an air bubble and eject the lens.

26.3 Suggested wearing schedules

The aim is to achieve a wearing time with hard lenses of 8–10 h by the time of the first aftercare check-up at about 2 weeks. This interval may be longer with soft lenses although all-day wear is often achieved more rapidly. The recommended schedule can be recorded as the starting time, increment and maximum.

Examples
Hard lenses: 3 + 1 . → 8 h
Previous failure: 1 + 1/2 → 8 h
PMMA: 1 + 1   → 8 h
                   or: 2 + 1/2 → 8 h
Low water content soft: 3 + 1   → 12 h
High water content soft: 4 + 2   → all day
Refits of hard with soft: 6 + 2   → all day

All-day wear is then achieved with hourly build-up if there are no contraindications at the first aftercare visit.

Practical advice

● The wearing schedules must be easy to understand and to follow.

● Advise the patient that, to avoid the risk of over-wear, the wearing schedule is a maximum and not a target.

● The total wearing time can be divided into two periods at different times of day, usually separated by a 4 h gap.

● Lenses should be removed and advice sought in the event of persistent discomfort, redness or other unusual symptoms.

26.4 General patient advice

New patients should not be allowed to wear lenses home because of the risk of early loss or damage. Before leaving, they should be given further clear instructions both verbally and in writing, covering the points outlined below.

Initial advice

- Lens identification.
- Wearing schedule.
- That lens comfort should be no worse than that already experienced on a tolerance trial and that the eyes should not become unduly red or sore.
- To bring to the first aftercare examination both the lens case and spectacles.
- That unless there is a serious problem with comfort or vision, they should come to the aftercare visit having worn lenses for as long as possible that particular day.
- The lens case, containing solution, should be carried at all times.

Lens care

- Method of lens storage (hard) or disinfection (soft).
- Not to change brand of solutions without first consulting the practitioner.
- Names of solutions equivalent to the original recommendations.
- The distinction between cleaning and disinfection.
- Never to use hard lens solutions with soft lenses and vice versa.
- That soft lenses are very fragile if they dry out, but are not necessarily spoiled since they recover after rehydration.
- To avoid placing two soft lenses in the same case compartment, because they may stick together and prove impossible to separate.

Unusual symptoms

- Sudden acute discomfort is probably caused by foreign bodies.

- Spectacle blur should not be experienced (except with PMMA).
- Some degree of adaptive photophobia is normal.
- Extreme environments in terms of temperature or humidity may affect both comfort and vision.
- Falling asleep with the lenses in or entering extreme environments may give temporary lens adhesion which may be released by the application of normal saline and gentle lid pressure.

Precautions

- Soft lenses should not be worn while eye drops or ointment are used for any reason (wait 1 h for drops and 4 h for ointment).
- Hard lenses could be worn with drops but not with ointment.
- Environments containing fumes, chemicals or sprays should be avoided.
- Traces of noxious chemicals must be very carefully removed from the hands before touching the lenses.
- To use goggles or photochromatic glasses for activities such as cycling or skiing to protect the eyes from wind, dust and dehydration.
- To take care with driving because of altered spatial judgement, and flare at night.
- When travelling or sunbathing to be careful not to fall asleep with lenses in, unless they are for extended wear.
- To avoid wearing lenses where possible on long flights because of the dry atmosphere on aircraft.
- Swimming is unwise with hard lenses because of the risk of loss. Soft lenses are often better but may still be lost; they might also cause stinging and red eyes if chlorine is absorbed into the material.

Chapter 27

Aftercare

27.1 First aftercare visit

The first aftercare examination should ideally take place after 2–3 weeks. If good progress has not been made by this time, success with the initial lenses is unlikely and significant changes may well need to be made. If the timing is too soon, nearly all patients complain of a multitude of genuinely adaptive symptoms; if too long after fitting, disturbing signs may have arisen or patients may have discontinued because of problems which are not adaptive.

The timing of aftercare appointments is important. Daily wear patients should be examined during the afternoon following several hours of contact lens use, whereas extended wear patients should be seen in the morning so that any overnight effects can be observed.

27.1.1 Initial discussion

Initial discussion should cover the following points which may require further assessment during the course of the examination:

- What progress the patient feels has been made.
- Are there any particular problems?
- Has the patient come in wearing the lenses – if not, why not?
- Maximum wearing time.
- Wearing time on the day of examination.
- Is handling satisfactory?
- Have all instructions been understood?
- Are instructions being followed?
- Are solutions being used correctly?
- Is the wearing schedule being followed?

- Are lenses being worn in the correct eye?
- Are soft lenses inside out?
- Is the patient in a happy and positive frame of mind?

Practical advice

- Carefully distinguish between visual and physical symptoms. Patients often complain of discomfort which really relates to vision.

27.1.2 Visual acuity and over-refraction

Snellen acuities are recorded monocularly and binocularly in the normal way. The quality of retinoscopy reflex is particularly important during assessment of vision and over-refraction (*see* Section 27.2).

27.1.3 Assessment of fitting with white light

White light examination either with low magnification or unaided gives a preliminary assessment of:

- Lens centration in primary position.
- Lens movement on blinking.
- Lens position with lateral and vertical eye movements.
- Blink rate.
- Completeness of blink.
- Conjunctival injection.
- Head position.
- Eye movements.
- Palpebral aperture.

Some of these factors may well be different during slit lamp examination where the head position is unnatural and light intensity much greater.

Practical advice

With a soft lens, movement is best seen by directing the beam from a hand-held pen torch, not necessarily from in front but from the side or below, so that the junction of the lenticular portion of the lens casts an easily observed annular light pattern and shadow onto the iris background. The movement of this is more easily discernible than that of the lens itself.

27.1.4 Assessment of fitting with fluorescein

Examination with fluorescein is mainly directed at hard lens fittings, although it can also be used with other specialized lenses such as silicone. Ultraviolet light does not give a useful assessment of fitting with hard lenses containing UV blockers (e.g. Boston RXD). High molecular weight fluorescein can be used with soft lenses, but generally adds little to white light observation. Fluorescein examination should reveal:

● The central fitting in respect of touch and clearance.

● Peripheral fitting and edge clearance.

● The speed of fluorescein mixing as an indicator of tear flow.

● 3 and 9 o'clock staining.

● Other areas of gross corneal staining or desiccation.

27.1.5 Slit lamp examination with lenses *in situ*

The slit-lamp is the major diagnostic instrument both at initial fitting and at all aftercare examinations. With lenses *in situ* it is used with varying degrees of magnification to check:

● Lens fit (centration and movement).

● Tear lens with slit beam.

● Signs of gross corneal oedema.

● The bulbar conjuctiva for signs of vessel irritation.

● The condition of lenses.

● Any air bubbles trapped under the lenses.

● Any debris trapped under the lenses.

● Wettability of lens surface

27.1.6. Supplementary procedures with lenses *in situ*

Supplementary procedures at this stage, with lenses still *in situ*, may include:

- Photography.
- Contrast sensitivity.
- Keratometry over front surface of lens (with soft).
- Placido disc or Klein keratoscope (with soft).

27.1.7 Slit lamp examination with lenses removed

Lenses are removed and ideally stored in the patient's own case. Fluorescein is then instilled and the eyes examined for:

- Any signs of corneal staining, noting both extent and depth.
- Any signs of corneal oedema (e.g. microcysts, striae), with both sclerotic scatter and direct observation.
- Corneal indentation (from sticking hard lenses).
- Scleral indentation (from tight soft lenses).
- Foreign bodies.
- Corneal desiccation.
- Qualitative assessment of tear film.
- Conjunctival injection or desiccation.
- Engorgement of limbal vessels.
- Irritation of lid margins.
- Changes to tarsal plate – seen with lid eversion.

27.1.8 Supplementary tests with lenses removed

Examination may indicate that supplementary procedures are advisable:

- Keratometry.
- Quantitative assessment of tear flow (*see* Section 3.6).
- Staining with rose bengal.
- Photography.
- Pachometry.
- Aesthesiometry.

27.1.9 Clinical adjustments or changes

The practitioner is now able to decide whether any symptoms are purely adaptive and can be temporarily ignored or whether some action is needed. There are several possible changes which may be necessary:

- Alteration to power or fitting. Hard and PMMA lenses may

be either modified or exchanged, depending upon the laboratory policy. Soft lenses require replacement.

● Refitting with the same general type of lens. For example, a hard lens with a higher *Dk* material; a soft lens with a different water content.

● Refitting with a totally different type of lens. For example, hard with soft; soft with hard; or spherical with toric.

● Different solutions. For example, completely changing the regimen because of allergy; adding saline as an extra rinsing solution; using a more efficient cleaner.

● Adjustment to the wearing schedule. Adaptation can often be helped with a change of wearing schedule, either slower or occasionally faster (e.g. to span a working day as soon as possible). A single period can be divided into two or vice versa.

27.1.10 Further discussion with the patient

The aftercare examination should conclude with further discussion, particularly to maintain patient enthusiasm. It should include:

● Reassurance concerning any subjective symptoms.

● Any lens change with reasons.

● Any changes to solutions regimen.

● Recommended date of next visit.

27.2 Visual problems

27.2.1 General factors

● First look for spherical errors and, if this improves acuity to a satisfactory level, small cylinders can be ignored.

● Distance acuity should be assessed separately from near and intermediate vision, since different and independent problems can arise.

● Snellen acuity is recorded in the usual way. Binocular acuity is often significantly better than that expected from monocular results. Contrast sensitivity measurements may explain visual problems where recorded acuities appear to be satisfactory.

● Retinoscopy reflex is an important diagnostic aid. It can show optical aberrations in a lens because of poor manufacture which may not be apparent with verification.

- A retinoscopy reflex improving after a blink with a soft lens indicates a tight fitting (*see* Chapter 16).

- The ophthalmoscope can also reveal lens aberrations as well as special features such as the position of a bifocal segment.

- Spectacle blur should not be present with hard and soft lenses. It is almost to be expected with PMMA.

DISTANCE VISION

Adaptive problems

- Variable vision. Most patients are affected to some degree during the early stages of adaptation.

- 'Foggy' vision due to greasy lenses. Usually worse in the afternoon and associated with poor blinking.

- Asthenopia, because of minor refractive changes or while the patient gets used to a different type of vision.

- Distorted vision. Myopes and hypermetropes notice, respectively, larger and smaller retinal image sizes.

- An apparently unequal change in over-refraction, with one eye requiring more minus and the other less, is a frequent indication that right and left lenses have been reversed.

Non-adaptive problems

- Blurred vision because of refractive changes. When tear flow has returned to normal, changes in refraction of 0.50 D can sometimes occur. An increase in minus may also indicate corneal oedema, so keratometry and slit lamp findings should also be assessed.

- Blurred vision because of residual astigmatism. This should be predictable at initial fitting, but is sometimes not observed until lenses have fully settled. Patients typically complain of ghosting. Consider a front surface toric.

- 'Foggy' vision because of greasy lenses. Tends to be worse immediately on insertion because of poor wetting or late in the day because of surface drying. Look for PC by everting the lids; this can sometimes occur within a few days of lens wear. Ensure solutions are being used correctly and possibly change to a different system. Hard lenses may need to be repolished and re-edged (sometimes necessary even with new lenses) or require an entirely different edge shape. Alternatively, consider a different lens material.

- Blurred vision because of oedema. Patients typically complain of 'foggy' or 'cloudy' vision. It can be differentiated from greasy deposits because if the lenses are cleaned and reinserted there is no temporary improvement in vision. It is much more common with PMMA, which should be fenestrated or refitted. Modern hard and soft lenses can be refitted with higher Dk materials.
- Asthenopia may be due to residual astigmatism, overcorrection, binocular imbalance or change in eye dominance (e.g. because of residual astigmatism in the dominant eye).

NEAR VISION

Near vision problems are frequently encountered in the early stages of adaptation with all types of lens (see Section 3.4).

INTERMEDIATE VISION

Music reading is a common problem because of the working distance, poor lighting conditions and instability of vision during adaptation. VDUs and painting can cause similar difficulties.

27.2.2 Hard and PMMA lenses

- Flare is worse with small PMMA lenses and flat peripheries. Possible modifications are thinning the mid-periphery or edges to improve centration. Otherwise fit a lens with a larger BOZD and total diameter; use less edge lift, especially in aspheric form; or change to a soft lens.
- Variable vision on blinking because of excessively mobile lenses.
- Blurred vision because of flexure. More common with hard than PMMA lenses. Consider a flatter fitting or greater centre thickness.

27.2.3 Soft lenses

- Flare is uncommon with soft lenses, but can occur with some designs of toric and with a displaced pupil. Where the patient cannot adapt, the lens should be remade with a larger FOZD or refitted with a different design.

- Blurred vision except after a blink suggests a tight fitting. This may be confirmed by the retinoscopy reflex.
- Variable vision, worse after a blink, suggests a loose fitting.
- Deterioration of vision during the course of the day may be due to lens dehydration.

27.3 Wearing problems

27.3.1 General factors

The practitioner must decide whether the fitting:

- Still looks as intended at the initial fitting. It is possible for either the eyes or the lenses to have altered.
- Is satisfactory in terms of position, movement, central fit, peripheral fit and centration.
- Is responsible for any subjective symptoms. Problems can arise, however satisfactory the fitting and quality of lens manufacture.
- Is causing any asymptomatic problems (e.g. oedema with an immobile lens).

27.3.2 Cornea

OEDEMA

Oedema is common with PMMA and quite feasible with hard and soft lenses where they are low riding, sticking, or the cornea has high oxygen requirements. Sclerotic scatter in a darkened room shows central oedema most clearly. This technique is not so successful with soft lenses, where the oedema tends to extend from limbus to limbus and may give rise to striae. Microcysts and bullae are other signs of corneal swelling. Subjectively, patients may complain of photophobia, cloudy vision or spectacle blur.

STAINING

Several types of staining are observed in practice.

Arcuate staining

Arcuate staining with hard lenses is usually found in the superior mid-periphery of the cornea (Figure 27.1). It is often asymptomatic and can be caused by:

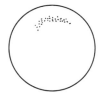

Figure 27.1 Arcuate staining

- Sharp transitions.
- Sharp or poorly finished edges.
- Insufficient edge lift.
- Sticking lens.
- Overall tight fitting.
- Tight lids giving excessive force during blinking.
- Badly finished or blocked fenestrations.
- Deposits on posterior lens surface.

'Pseudo-arcuate' staining is sometimes observed with narrow edge lift. The lens periphery gives an arcuate pressure effect which does not actually take up fluorescein stain. It is sometimes sufficient to reveal the Fischer–Schweitzer corneal mosaic.

Remedies to arcuate staining include:

- Fully blending all transitions.
- Re-edging.
- Increasing edge lift.
- Reducing BOZD.
- Flatter BOZR.
- Changing to a different total diameter.

Arcuate staining is also observed with both daily and extended wear soft lenses. Although it can occur in most regions of the cornea, it is more commonly found towards the superior limbus with thicker and higher water content lenses. It has been referred to as superior epithelial arcuate lesions (SEALS) [1] and usually causes discomfort with reduced wearing time, particularly when associated with corneal drying. In severe cases there is gradually advancing superior vascularization. It is usually resolved by changing the design or water content, but may occasionally necessitate refitting with hard lenses.

3 and 9 o'clock staining

3 and 9 o'clock staining is created by drying in the nasal and temporal areas of the cornea (Figure 27.2). It is a more frequent

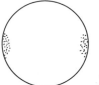

Figure 27.2 3 and 9 o'clock staining

problem with hard lenses than with PMMA, with several possible causes. These must be recognized before the correct remedial action can be taken:

● Poor blinking.

● Inadequate tear film.

● Wide palpebral apertures.

● Periphery too flat or edges too thick (lid held away from the corneal surface – 'lid gap').

● Periphery too tight (physical disruption of tear film).

● Total diameter too large (physical disruption of tear film).

● Total diameter too small (disincentive to proper blinking).

● The hard lens material (tear film disrupted by surface wetting properties).

It may be resolved by:

● Correct blinking.

● A thinner lens.

● Refitting with a lid attachment design (*see* Section 6.5).

● A different total diameter.

● A different lens periphery.

● Refitting with moulded CAB or PMMA.

● Refitting with soft lenses.

Central staining
Central staining is caused by the breakdown of the corneal epithelium as a result of corneal oedema (Figure 27.3). It is possible with any type of lens, but is usually associated with PMMA.

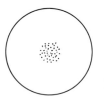

Figure 27.3 Central staining

Punctate staining (corneal stippling)

Punctate staining may be either intense or diffuse and has a variety of causes:

- Corneal desiccation between the lower periphery of a hard lens and the limbus due to exposure of the epithelium where it is not lubricated by the lids on blinking (Figure 27.4). It may be regarded as a more superficial and more diffuse type of 3 and 9 o'clock staining and responds to the same remedial actions.

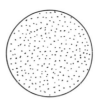

Figure 27.4 Inferior punctate staining

Figure 27.5 Diffuse punctate staining

- Solutions. Punctates vary from extremely fine and diffuse over the entire corneal surface with no apparent symptoms (Figure 27.5), to large coalescent areas with gross hyperaemia, lacrimation and discomfort.
- Material allergies.
- Toxic reactions (e.g. to contaminated soft lenses or unreacted monomers in hard lenses).

Foreign body

Staining is typically superficial and linear with a curved or zigzag shape (Figure 27.6), although sometimes a foreign body (FB) may be trapped by the lens deep into the cornea. Sudden sharp FB pain is a constant minor hazard with hard lenses and, because the corneal sensitivity is not depressed to the same extent as PMMA, often causes greater problems.

Figure 27.6 Foreign body tracks

Irregular staining

Irregular staining may have a variety of possible causes:

- Poorly fitting lens.
- Damaged lens.
- Deposits on posterior lens surface.
- Badly finished or blocked fenestration.

Air bubbles (dimpling)

Dimpling occurs mainly with hard lenses, but is also possible with soft. The small air bubbles trapped in a pool of tears beneath a contact lens act as foreign bodies. They give a fairly dramatic appearance with fluorescein, but do not give true staining (Figure 27.7). If the lens is removed and the eye rinsed

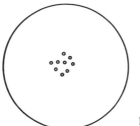

Figure 27.7 Central dimpling

with saline, irregular depressions can be seen in the corneal surface, but the apparent staining disappears with no actual uptake of fluorescein by the epithelium. Dimpling causes no discomfort, but gives blurred vision if it occurs within the pupil area where it is easily detected with both the retinoscope and ophthalmoscope. As the bubbles coalesce, they can either froth or occasionally form a single large bubble which may lead to corneal desiccation.

Dimpling is found:

- Centrally, with a steep fitting.
- Superiorly, under a flat periphery in a stable high-riding lens.
- With keratoconus and other irregular corneas.

It can be helped by:

- Loosening the fit to promote better tear flow.
- Changing the BOZD or total diameter.
- Fenestration, although this could make it worse.

Practical advice

Small, discrete areas of staining and isolated punctates can often be safely ignored with hard lenses. Much more careful assessment is necessary with soft lenses to ensure that they are not a precursor to more serious corneal complication.

27.3.3 Limbus

BLOOD VESSELS

It is always important to examine carefully the superior corneoscleral junction, since the limbal blood vessels dilate in response to any adverse stimulus such as physical irritation, insufficient oxygen or solutions reaction. It is also possible for 'ghost' vessels from previous contact lens wear to refill within a few days if stimulated by these same factors.

STAINING

Staining at the limbus can occur for various reasons:

● Solutions reaction
● Abrasions from lens edges.
● Desiccation (3 and 9 o'clock).
● Inferior, because of exposure.
● Hypoxia beneath the upper lid.

DELLEN

The long-term consequence of severe 3 and 9 o'clock desiccation with hard and PMMA lenses is dellen formation. This shows as marked corneal thinning at the limbus associated with severe conjunctival injection. Recovery, however, can occur within a few days on ceasing contact lens wear.

LIMBAL OPACIFICATION

Although limbal opacification is usually a long-term response to PMMA, it can occur more rapidly with modern hard lenses. It is observed together with an advancing area of corneal drying, and on rare occasions it is observed by the time of the first aftercare examination.

Pingueculae may become injected during contact lens wear, particularly where associated with poor blinking and dry eyes. Patients often notice them for the first time when beginning to use contact lenses and may require reassurance that they are benign and are not actually caused by the lenses.

27.3.4 Bulbar conjunctiva

INJECTION

Some minor degree of redness is frequently adaptive and there may be staining with either fluorescein or rose bengal. More severe conjunctival injection can be due to:

- Solutions reaction.
- Other allergies.
- Poor blinking.
- 3 and 9 o'clock staining.
- Other desiccation.
- Infections.
- Physical irritation.

27.3.5 Lids

PAPILLARY CONJUNCTIVITIS

Papillary conjunctivitis (PC) is an inflammation of the papillary conjunctiva of, usually, the upper lids, characterized by the presence of irregularly shaped papillae. These may appear similar to those found with vernal catarrh, but are histologically different and progress in four distinct stages [2]:

(1) Preclinical stage with mild increase in mucus production.

(2) Conjunctival hyperaemia and thickening with slight elevation of normal papillae. Vascular tufts can be seen in the papillae.

(3) Formation of larger papillae from coalescent smaller papillae, often starting from the inner and outer canthi.

(4) Formation of elevated, giant papillae with flattened heads which can stain with fluorescein.

Contact lens wearers are usually seen at stages (1) or (2). The symptoms are quite distinctive:

- Itching on lens removal.
- Discharge in the morning, typically yellow in colour.
- Severe lens deposits causing blurred vision.
- Excessive movement of the lens which is pulled by the rough surface of the upper lid.
- Gradually deteriorating comfort.

The condition can be either unilateral or bilateral and, although more typically a problem of soft lens wear, can be found with all lens types. There are several causative factors, working either on their own or in conjunction:

- Allergic response to the lens material.
- Auto-immune allergic response to protein deposits on the lens surface.
- Solutions sensitivity.
- Mechanical irritation.
- Environmental irritation.
- Predisposition with atopic patients (e.g. hay fever sufferers).

Resolving PC may require several courses of action:

- Consider medical referral for treatment with either sodium cromoglycate 2% (Opticrom) or steroids such as Predsol-n.
- Discontinue lens wear for possibly up to 3 months.
- Discontinue extended wear, at least until condition is resolved.
- Fit new soft lenses or repolish hard.
- Fit new soft lenses before the hay fever season.
- Ensure regular lens replacement.
- Eliminate all preserved solutions.
- Change to a peroxide system.
- Ensure regular use of enzyme tablets.
- With soft lenses, consider a different material or refitting with hard.

● With hard lenses, avoid silicone acrylates and consider CAB or fluoropolymers.

MISCELLANEOUS LID PROBLEMS

Ther are several minor lid problems. The majority are unconnected with contact lenses, although patients may require reassurance of this point.

● Concretions.
● Make-up trapped on palpebral conjunctiva.
● Blocked meibomian glands and frothing at lid margin.
● Styes and cysts.
● Blepharitis exacerbated by contact lens wear.
● Vesicles on lid margins.
● Skin allergies, often caused by make-up but sometimes by solutions.
● Lid spasms and twitching.

27.3.6 Lens adhesion

Adhesion has been regarded as a hard lens extended wear problem (see Section 20.5). It is not uncommon, however, with daily wear towards the end of the day. Patients are often asymptomatic, but the possible problems are:

● Arcuate staining.
● Redness.
● Trapped debris.
● Corneal distortion.
● Infection.

Lens adhesion can be caused by a variety of factors:

● Dry eyes.
● Tight lids.
● Periphery too narrow.
● Lens material (more common with CAB).
● Lens design (more common with aspheric lenses).

It is helped by:

● Flattening the periphery.

- Changing the material.
- Improved blinking.
- Lubricating drops.

27.3.7 Environmental and general factors

Some of the most difficult problems are caused not by the lenses but by the environment or external factors:

- Central heating.
- Air conditioning.
- Low humidity.
- High altitude.
- Staring at VDU screens.
- Polluted atmospheres.
- Poor lighting.

Symptoms of discomfort are exacerbated by other factors:

- Alcohol.
- Diet.
- Systemic drugs (see Section 28.3).
- Oral contraceptives.
- Tiredness.
- Poor general health.
- Pregnancy.
- Psychological effects of tension.

27.3.8 Blinking

Infrequent or incomplete blinking is a particular difficulty with hard and PMMA lenses. It causes several problems:

- Oedema because of insufficient tear pump.
- 3 and 9 o'clock staining.
- Other corneal and conjunctival desiccation.
- Conjunctival injection.
- General discomfort.
- Lens deposits and blurred vision.

Incomplete blinking with soft lenses also causes problems such as inferior corneal staining because of dehydration and lens deposits.

Practical advice

Hard lenses act as a strong disincentive to correct blinking, so retraining is rarely successful. Refitting with soft lenses is often the best solution.

27.4 Aftercare routine for yearly or longer intervals

Examination after 12 months or a longer period is especially concerned with the possible long-term consequences of contact lens wear and the condition of the lenses. It includes the same stages as the first aftercare routine (*see* Sections 27.1.1 to 27.1.10) with the key additions of:

- Reassessment of contact lens refraction and fitting with trial lenses.
- Spectacle refraction (*see* Section 28.4).
- Ophthalmoscopy – this may be the only opportunity for fundus and ophthalmic examination.
- Assessment of contact lens condition.

27.4.1 Ocular examination

CORNEA

- Vascularization or neovascularization.
- Oedematous responses (microcysts, bullae, striae).
- Signs of infection (nummular or other infiltrates).
- Corneal thinning.
- Endothelial polymegathism.
- Chronic staining.

CONJUNCTIVA

- Desiccation.

- Injection.
- Pingueculae.

LIDS

- Position.
- PC.
- Concretions.
- Patency of meibomian glands.

TEARS

- Qualitative assessment.
- Break-up time.

OVER-REFRACTION

- Comparison with previously recorded acuities.
- Change in myopia or hypermetropia.
- Change in astigmatism.

27.4.2 Other factors

REASSESSING CONTACT LENS REFRACTION AND FITTING

Old and deposited lenses frequently give reduced acuity. Hard lenses may have distorted with repeated handling and soft become less flexible with age. Spurious refractive changes of up to 1.00 D can be found, so it is essential to reassess both refractive result and fitting with fresh trial lenses (preferably the original) in order to obtain a reliable result.

ASSESSING CONTACT LENS CONDITION

It is also important to examine the lens condition both on the eye with the slit lamp and off the eye with a projection microscope. These instruments allow easy demonstration to the patient of surface and edge defects or signs of ageing (*see* Section 28.5).

SOLUTIONS

It is important to establish that the patient is using solutions correctly. Common errors are:

- Changing brands without consulting the practitioner.
- Omitting to use a daily cleaner.
- Insufficient rinsing of cleaning solution.
- Forgetting to use enzyme tablets.
- Using preserved instead of unpreserved saline.
- Thinking saline is a storage and disinfection solution.
- Forgetting to add the disinfection tablet with chlorine systems.

References

1. Hine, N., Back, A. and Holden, B.A. (1987) Aetiology of arcuate epithelial lesions induced by hydrogels. *Transactions of the British Contact Lens Association Annual Clinical Conference*, **4**, 48–50.
2. Allansmith, M.R., Korb, D.R., Freiner, J.V., Henriquez, A.S., Simon, M.A. and Finnemore, V.M. (1977) Giant papillary conjunctivitis in contact lens wearers. *American Journal of Ophthalmology*, **83**, 697–708.

Chapter 28

Supplementary aftercare

28.1 Emergencies

Emergencies, either perceived or real, are a fairly routine occurrence in contact lens practice. It is a common assumption by patients that the lenses are the invariable cause of any ocular problem and it may require all of the practitioner's skill to differentiate between contact lens and non-contact lens emergencies.

Overwear syndrome (acute epithelial necrosis; 3 a.m. syndrome)

This is commonly associated with PMMA, although not unknown with either hard or soft lenses. The patient is typically awakened in the middle of the night with extreme pain ('red hot needles' is the usual description), photophobia and lacrimation. It is an extreme response to gross corneal oedema as a result of excessive contact lens wear. Typical causes are:

- Too fast initial wearing schedule.
- Patient forgetting to remove lenses at a specified time.
- All-day use after a gap in lens wear because of loss.
- Falling asleep with lenses in.
- Chronic oedema with longer than normal wear in a hot and stuffy atmosphere.

Examination, where feasible, shows large areas of corneal staining. Treatment may well require local anaesthetic, antibiotic to minimize the risk of secondary infection, and 'pad and bandaging' in a darkened room for 24 h. The epithelium usually recovers within two or three days, although contact lens wear should not be resumed for at least a week and not until the practitioner has confirmed that the cornea is clear. A very slow wearing schedule is then indicated. Patients require considerable reassurance that they will not suffer permanent damage to their eyes.

Practical advice

Local anaesthetics tend to retard epithelial healing and should only be used in cases of extreme pain. The preferred analgesic is often aspirin with whisky.

Foreign bodies

These are much more common with hard and PMMA lenses. The damage to the corneal epithelium, however, can sometimes be greater with soft lenses because the foreign body remains trapped behind the lens for a longer period of time. Patients complain of sudden, acute pain during the wearing day. The lens must be removed and fluorescein instilled to assess the depth of staining with slit lamp optic section. Treatment consists of antibiotic, with 'pad and bandaging' in extreme cases.

Corneal abrasions

Similar symptoms to foreign bodies are found with severe abrasions. These may be caused by poor lens handling; inserting or wearing damaged lenses; lenses breaking in the eye; and fitting problems.

Infections

Infections may be either connected or unconnected with contact lens wear. Immediate medical treatment is particularly required for corneal ulcers to minimize any risk of permanent visual loss.

Solutions problems

A high proportion of soft lens emergencies relate to solutions reactions. Careful questioning is sometimes necessary to reveal either patient error or the offending solution. Typical problems are:

- Genuine allergic responses.
- Using hard lens solutions with soft lenses.
- Not neutralizing lenses stored in hydrogen peroxide.
- Confusing soaking and cleaning solutions.

- Reaction to enzyme tablets.
- Adverse reaction after intensive cleaning.
- Using preserved comfort drops in an otherwise non-preserved regimen.
- Using preserved therapeutic drops.
- Patients changing to a brand different from that originally recommended by the practitioner.
- Patients being sold an incorrect solution.

Contaminated lenses

This mainly applies to soft lenses contaminated by products like paint, varnish, hair-spray and make-up, either by direct contact or indirectly via the hands. Hard lenses are occasionally affected.

'Red eye'

The 'red eye' reaction typically occurs with soft extended wear lenses (*see* Section 20.4.2) as gross unilateral hyperaemia, associated with varying degrees of pain, photophobia, lacrimation and limbal infiltrates.

28.2 Grief cases

Not all patients adapt well to contact lenses, however carefully they are fitted. This may be due to the practitioner, the patient or limitations in available lens designs [1].

28.2.1 Causes

The main reasons for grief cases wishing to consult another practitioner are:

- Poor vision or comfort because of fitting or refitting with the wrong type of lens.
- Wearing the correct type of lens but an unsatisfactory fitting.
- Poor vision or comfort because of badly manufactured lenses.
- Using inappropriate solutions.
- Recurrent deposits or greasy lenses.

- Red eyes or 3 and 9 o'clock staining because of poor blinking.
- Dry eyes.
- Spectacle blur.
- Allergic response to materials or solutions.
- The patient does not understand or follow instructions.
- The presence of an eye infection, either connected or unconnected with the contact lenses.
- The patient may no longer be suitable for contact lens wear because of corneal exhaustion, dry eyes or environmental factors.
- The patient has never really been suitable for contact lenses.
- The patient may have lost confidence in the previous practitioner, although the lenses are perfectly satisfactory.

28.2.2 Courses of action

The new practitioner must decide on the main reason for previous dissatisfaction and whether successful contact lens wear is feasible. The following are the most common courses of action:

- Modify existing lenses. This applies mainly to PMMA and hard lenses.
- Refit lenses of the same general type (e.g. soft with soft or hard with hard), but use a different material, Dk or design.
- Refit with lenses of an altogether different type (e.g. soft with hard or hard with soft).
- Change the solutions or disinfection system. This is often advisable, even where refitting is also carried out.
- Give advice on correct blinking.
- Give clear instructions in the correct use of solutions, even where there is no sensitivity problem.
- Give correct instructions in lens handling and maintenance.
- Refer for medical opinion.
- Advise patients that they are now unsuitable for lenses. They will be disappointed, but at the same time accept the fact that they have at last been given unequivocal advice.

Practical advice

- Grief cases have generally been disillusioned with contact lenses and are seeking a swift and positive resolution to their problems.
- Where refitting is necessary, dispense lenses from stock.
- Give a safe but rapid wearing schedule.
- Put a time limit of 2–3 weeks on any course of action to prevent an unsuccessful case dragging on interminably.
- Where only partial success is possible, advise patients to be realistic, accept a restricted wearing time or discontinue.

28.2.3 Avoiding grief cases

- Do not refit lenses just for the sake of it. If a patient is entirely happy with existing lenses and examination reveals no serious, asymptomatic problems (e.g. corneal oedema or vascularization), then leave well alone.
- Explain, nevertheless, any relevant new developments and clarify misconceptions (e.g. disposables are not appropriate for toric hard lens wearers).
- Do not refit PMMA wearers with soft lenses (see Chapter 13).
- If a patient has been refitted with theoretically better lenses (e.g. PMMA with hard or low water content soft with high) and they do not settle rapidly, then return to the previous type without delay.
- If a replacement lens does not settle rapidly with an experienced lens wearer, change it or refit.
- Use only the best possible quality lenses. Poorly made lenses can waste considerable practitioner time.
- Adopt a flexible and open-minded approach to contact lens fitting and be prepared to change from one type to another if problems arise.

28.3 Side effects of systemic drugs

Many systemic drugs have side effects which give rise to symptoms of discomfort, blurred vision, dryness and lens discoloration (Table 28.1).

Table 28.1 Systemic drugs and their side effects

Drug	Side effect
CENTRAL NERVOUS SYSTEM	
Carbamazepine (Tegretol)	Conjunctivitis and photophobia
Maprotiline (Ludiomil)	Intolerance to contact lenses and loss of tear fluid
Diazepam (Valium)	Lowered visual acuity and reduced tear production
Dothiepin (Prothiaden)	Reduced tear flow
Amitriptyline (Tryptizol)	Reduced tear flow
Lorazepam (Atavan)	Dry eye
BLOOD PRESSURE AND HEART CONDITIONS	
Atenolol (Tenormin) / Isosorbide (Binitrat)	Smarting eyes and diffuse conjunctival injection with very dry eyes
Amiodarone (Cordarone)	Faint striae in both corneas and yellow brown deposits
Oxprenolol (Trasidrex)	Dry eye/conjunctivitis
Cyclopenthiazide	Dry eye/conjunctivitis
Methyldopa (Aldomet)	Keratoconjunctivitis sicca
MUSCULOSKELETAL DISORDERS (ANTI-INFLAMMATORY)	
Penicillamine (Distamine)	Dry eye and reduced vision
URINARY ANTI-INFECTIVES	
Trimethoprim / Sulphamethoxazole (Septrin)	Dryness and irritation
Nitrofurantoin (Furadantin)	Marked irritation with profuse lacrimation
ANTI-OBESITY	
Diethylpropion (Tenuate Dospan)	Reduced tear production and over-wear syndrome
ANTI-ALLERGIC	
Sodium cromoglycate (Opticrom)	Reduced tear production
ANTIBIOTICS	
Doxycycline (Vibramycin)	Marked photophobia and contact lens sensitivity
RESPIRATORY SYSTEM	
Beclomethasone (Becotide) / Salbutamol (Ventolin)	Increased sensitivity to contact lenses and solutions
Rifampicin (for TB)	Discolours soft lenses yellow
ORAL CONTRACEPTIVE	
Levonorgestrel (Microval)	Increase in astigmatism
Ovranette	Reduced tolerance to contact lenses
ALIMENTARY SYSTEM	
Sulphasalazine (for Crohn's disease)	Discolours soft lenses
NASAL DECONGESTANTS	
Brompheniramine / Phenylephrine	Reduced tolerance to soft contact lens wear
Adrenaline (epinephrine)	Discolours soft lenses
ANTIHISTAMINES	
Piriton / Triludan	Dehydration

Practical advice

- Pathologies of the cornea due to side effects are serious and tend to be progressive as the dosage continues.
- Use the yellow card system to report any adverse response to either contact lens products or systemic drugs.

28.4 Prescribing spectacles for contact lens wearers

The factors to consider include:

- Establishing the correct Rx.
- Providing a correction which is visually comfortable.
- Time of examination.
- When the spectacles are likely to be worn.
- Type of contact lens worn.

Non-tolerances are a frequent problem because, irrespective of contact lens type, many patients find great difficulty in adapting to the different nature of a spectacle correction worn in front of rather than on the eye. Typical problems are:

- Visual distortion (e.g. sloping floors and bowed door frames).
- Different spatial perspective.
- Different image size.
- Restricted field of view.
- Reflections, especially at night.
- Intolerance to full correction.
- Intolerance to cylinders.

Typical causes are:

- No spectacle refraction for several years and a correction showing a very marked increase in myopia.
- Astigmatism very different in axis and power compared with any previous correction.
- Patients may literally have worn no spectacles for decades because with PMMA it was not feasible to obtain a satisfactory result.

● Contact lens monovision (deliberate or accidental) may give difficulty with either bifocals or separate distance and near spectacles.

Practical advice

● Explain the potential problems to the patient.
● Take notice of any pre-contact lens spectacles, however old.
● Give maximum possible binocular addition.
● Consider under-correcting spheres by 0.25–0.50 D.
● Consider under-correcting or omitting cylinders.
● Be careful not to change eye dominance.
● Repeat refraction on another occasion if it does not correlate with the contact lenses, keratometry and previous correction.

28.4.1 PMMA

Long-term PMMA wearers are the most difficult for prescribing spectacles because:

● There is almost invariably some degree of corneal distortion or moulding.
● There is frequently some level of corneal oedema.
● Refraction often gives a poor and unreliable end-point.
● Acuity may be depressed.

The main problem, however, is that after PMMA lenses have been removed, the refraction continuously changes for several weeks while the corneal curvature is undergoing an equivalent cycle of change. Although there are wide individual differences, there is an average decrease in myopia of 1.32 D over the first 3 days, followed by an increase in myopia up to 21 days (Figure 28.1) [2]. At the same time, there is a strong trend towards increased with-the-rule astigmatism.

In practical terms, therefore, there is no merit whatever in leaving out lenses for periods of several days. Not only is it extremely inconvenient for the patients, especially if they are highly myopic with no current spectacles, but it is also liable to

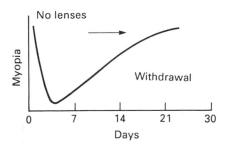

Figure 28.1 Myopia after PMMA lens removal (Rengstorff, 1967)

give a wildly inaccurate result. The once common advice of removing lenses for two or three days before refraction, in fact gives an examination time at the point of maximum change.

There are two realistic times for examination, the choice of which should be discussed with the patient according to when the correction is to be used:

(1) Afternoon, immediately on removal of lenses, gives the closest approximation to a correction for use in the evenings when lenses have been removed for the day.
(2) Morning, prior to insertion of lenses, simulates the occasion when contact lenses will not be worn for a day.

The morning result is usually 0.50–0.75 D less. Undercorrecting the evening refraction can often give a satisfactory compromise.

28.4.2 Hard lenses

Most modern hard lenses cause few problems compared with PMMA, but some degree of corneal moulding may be encountered, particularly with astigmatic eyes and where aspheric designs are used. Pronounced distortion occurs in cases of lens adhesion, and refraction should be postponed.

Satisfactory refraction is usually achieved immediately on removal of lenses. If the result does not correlate with the contact lenses, keratometry and any previous spectacles, it should be repeated as a morning refraction.

Where PMMA has been refitted with hard lenses, wait about 2 months before refracting for spectacles, by which time most corneal changes will have resolved. This is confirmed by monitoring 'K' readings.

28.4.3 Soft lenses

Corneal curvature and refractive changes are far less common with soft lenses, although some steepening of the vertical meridian may occur. There is little mechanical moulding, and where oedema is present it generally extends from limbus to limbus without localized changes in curvature or physical distortion. Refraction on removal of soft lenses generally gives a good result, but where there is any doubt it should be repeated in the morning.

28.5 Lens ageing

28.5.1 Soft lenses

Soft lenses stored in sealed vials remain in good condition for several years, but once they are worn regularly lens deterioration occurs in a variety of ways. Unlike hard lenses, ageing is a common cause of lens replacement influenced by a variety of factors:

- Lens material. High water content lenses deteriorate more rapidly than HEMA because of deposits and discolouration.

- Wearing schedule. Extended wear lenses are more badly affected by deposits than those used daily.

- Tear chemistry. Some patients' lenses last only a few weeks, whereas others can remain in acceptable condition for several years. Dry eyes cause particular problems.

- Method of disinfection. Lenses have a shorter life span when sterilized by heat compared with solutions. Hydrogen peroxide is particularly good at keeping lenses in optimum condition (*see* Section 25.4).

- Regularity and method of cleaning.

- Patient care.

- The environment in which lenses are worn. Dry atmospheres enhance lens deposits.

Protein deposits

All lenses suffer protein deposits to some extent. With HEMA, in particular, there is a chemical bonding between tear protein and the polymer's hydroxyl groups [3]. Heat disinfection exacerbates the problem by denaturing any surface protein which has not been removed by proper cleaning. It is observed as a blue-grey film by oblique illumination against a dark background (dark-field illumination). It can also be seen during slit lamp examination if the patient stares and the lens surface is allowed to dry.

Discolouration

Most high water content lenses suffer from brown discoloration to some extent. HEMA can also be affected and heat aggravates the problem. Adrenaline compounds in the tears, nicotine and make-up have been suggested as other causes. Some lenses fluoresce with ultraviolet light. This effect may be due either to the material (with new lenses) or chlorhexidine bound to surface deposits. Acuity may be reduced and significant reductions in light transmission occur [4,5]. Hormonal problems and systemic drugs have also been implicated (see Section 28.3).

White spots

White spots almost invariably occur on the front surface of the lens. In the early stages they appear as fine punctate dots and gradually develop into discrete, elevated deposits scattered irregularly within the area of the exposed palpebral aperture. High water content lenses and those for extended wear are much more affected, particularly with dry-eyed patients and poor blinkers. In severe cases, white spots can be over 1 mm across and extremely uncomfortable. These larger deposits have also been referred to as 'mulberries' and 'jelly-bumps'. The composition of white spots has been variously described as a combination of mucoprotein and lipids; mucopolysaccharides; and calcium phosphate and calcium carbonate [6].

Rust spots

Rust spots are mainly due to atmospheric pollution and are more often observed in patients from industrial areas or who travel by train. They are a form of benign ferrous contamination affecting all types of soft lens and are occasionally found as a manufacturing fault [7].

Surface and edge deterioration

As lenses become older and less flexible, they become uncomfortable because of surface scratches and edge chips. Engravings can either crack or become encrusted with deposits. Uneven drying of protein film at the lens periphery can cause crenellated edges.

Fitting changes

Lenses with deposits are more influenced by the upper lid and significant changes in fitting characteristics can occur. Usually they become looser and corneal diameter lenses may become badly decentred. High riding lenses are frequently associated with PC where the irregular tarsal plate pulls the deposited lens out of position.

Refractive changes

Old and less flexible lenses frequently give reduced acuity as well as spurious changes in over-refraction of as much as 1.00 D. The lens power, therefore, should always be rechecked with a fresh trial lens when refitting is necessary.

Practical advice

- Before undertaking professional cleaning, advise patients that it will be carried out 'at their own risk'. Unpredictable and irreversible changes can occur to lens dimensions.
- A small minority of highly allergic patients can produce a severe reaction to professionally cleaned lenses.
- Use a shorter cleaning time and lower temperature with high water content lenses.
- Protein film and discolouration can usually be removed or improved by professional cleaning.
- White spots do not respond well and lenses may fail to survive intensive cleaning.
- It is sometimes beneficial to leave lenses in hydrogen peroxide for up to a week, changing the solution every two or three days, before intensive cleaning with a product like Liprofin.
- Lenses with cracks and chips harbour micro-organisms and should be replaced.

- Patients should be encouraged to replace lenses on a regular basis, rather than expect an unrealistically long life span.

___

28.5.2 Hard lenses

Hard lenses do not deteriorate in the same way as soft lenses. Their life span is approximately 2–4 years but, depending upon material, they do deteriorate in various ways.

Deposits

Silicone acrylate materials (*see* Chapter 5) attract protein from the tears and most patients benefit from the use of enzyme tablets. Monthly soaking is usually sufficient, although some patients require more frequent treatment.

Fluorosilicone acrylates present less of a problem with protein and many of the materials do not require enzyme tablets.

CAB lenses do not contain silicone. Protein deposits are rarely a problem and enzyme tablets are almost always unnecessary. Lenses do attract lipids, however, so greasing is sometimes a problem.

Discolouration

Discolouration is rarely a problem with most materials. However, some – even when new – show haziness and lack of optical transparency. CAB lenses may also become hazy after 12–18 months.

Surface and edge deterioration

Some of the fluorosilicone acrylates have proved quite brittle, and edge damage or complete breakage are not uncommon. Certain of the high *Dk* silicone acrylates suffer from surface crazing. CAB lenses are more prone to surface scratching.

28.5.3 PMMA

PMMA is still the most stable and inert material. It attracts little in the way of permanent deposits, although some patients are troubled by greasing with older or scratched lenses. It can readily be repolished and frequently gives a life span in excess of five years.

28.6 Lens modification

Modifications may be found necessary either during initial adaptation or at annual aftercare examinations. Adjustments are usually better left to the laboratory, especially with the less stable modern hard lenses. There are some occasions, however, when it is essential for lenses to be modified on the spot, and the following minimum equipment should be available:

● Drum with motorized spindle.
● Velveteen pad.
● Reversible suction holder or chuck.
● Selection of convex radius tools with polishing tape.
● Polishing medium (X Pal for hard and Silvo for PMMA lenses).

28.6.1 Hard and PMMA lenses

It is possible to make the following modifications:

● Blend and flatten peripheral radii.
● Reduce TD.
● Minor changes to BVP.
● Repolish or reshape edges.
● Repolish front surfaces.
● Fenestration.
● Truncation.

Practical advice

● Ensure the pad or tool is wet at all times.
● All modifications tend to make the fit looser.
● It is not feasible to tighten the fit by modification.
● Do not attempt to modify surface-treated lenses.
● Modern hard lens materials require greater care to avoid distortion and far less pressure than PMMA.

Blending and flattening of peripheral curves

- The lens is held centrally by the convex surface with a suction holder or negative chuck.
- A tape-covered convex tool of the required radius is selected.
- The lens is rotated against the tool in the opposite direction of motion to the spindle.

Changing the BVP

It is easier to add minus than plus power without upsetting the image quality. The limits for successful modification are about $-0.75\,\mathrm{D}$ and $+0.50\,\mathrm{D}$ for hard lenses; $-1.00\,\mathrm{D}$ and $+0.75\,\mathrm{D}$ for PMMA.

Plus power

The lens is mounted centrally by the concave surface with a suction holder or long-stemmed chuck. It is held against the centre of a velveteen pad moistened with polish and gently rocked, working from periphery to centre.

Negative power

The lens is pressed with one finger against a stationary pad, well oiled with polish. It is rotated in small circles about 10 times clockwise and then anticlockwise, working from centre to periphery. This adds about $-0.25\,\mathrm{D}$ and is repeated for more minus.

Polishing the edges

The lens is attached to a strong suction holder or chuck and the edge rocked and rotated against a well-oiled, spinning pad.

Polishing the surface

The lens is mounted as if for adding positive power, but also drawn across the pad. This adds minus to neutralize any power change. After two passes, both the surface and focimeter image are checked.

28.6.2 Scleral lenses

Possible modifications:

- Back optic grind-out.
- Transitional grind-out.
- Fenestration.
- Channelling.
- BVP.
- Back scleral size reduction.

References

1. Gasson, A.P. (1984) Aftercare – the good, the bad and the ugly. *Transactions of the British Contact Lens Association Annual Clinical Conference*, **7**, 143–145
2. Rengstorff, R.H. (1967) Variations in myopia measurements: an after-effect observed with habitual wearers of contact lenses. *American Journal of Optometry*, **44**, 149–161
3. Cummings, J.S. (1973) The future of soft contact lenses. *Manufacturing Optics International*, **26**, 309–312
4. Gasson, A.P. (1975) Visual considerations with hydrophilic lenses. *Ophthalmic Optician*, **15**, 439–448
5. Ganju, S.N. and Cordrey, P. (1976) Removal of adsorbed preservative in soft contact lenses. *Optician*, **171**(4423), 16, 18, 20–21
6. Ruben, M., Triparthi, R.C. and Winder, A.F. (1975) Calcium deposition as a cause of spoilation of hydrophilic soft contact lenses. *British Journal of Ophthalmology*, **59**, 141–148
7. Loran, D.F.C. (1973) Surface corrosion of hydrogel contact lenses. *Contact Lens*, **4**, 3–10

Chapter 29

Contact lenses and children

29.1 Management

29.1.1 Parental management

Sympathetic management is essential, because parents are naturally concerned about eye problems which become evident within a few weeks of birth, whether the treatment is surgery or simply optical correction. Ametropic children as young as 4 or 5 years may be brought in for contact lenses because the parents cannot accept the idea of spectacles. A contact lens trial may help appreciation of vision where children have reacted against spectacles.

29.1.2 Child management

Babies are easy to manage as no communication is necessary, whereas infants need the stimulation of toys to help with attention. Children of 5 years and older need a great deal of patience and kindness at the initial fitting, for the essential

Table 29.1 Approximate corneal dimensions for children*

	Keratometry (mm)	Corneal diameter (mm)
Baby (? month old)	6.90	10.0
Infant (4 years old)	7.60	11.0

*Adult dimensions are reached at approximately 10 years of age.

building up of confidence. Apart from fear of the unknown, they are disturbed by the manipulation necessary for insertion and removal and can be frightened of the optical equipment. Keratometry and slit lamp examination can be performed from an early age with a co-operative child, who can be held by the parent, kneel on a stool or stand at the instrument.

29.2 Refractive applications

29.2.1 Myopia

The correction of high myopia may improve both acuity and the field of view. Near vision develops without any optical correction. The first choice is often soft, but the thick edge of a high minus lens may lead to vascularization in the long term.

Hard materials of medium Dk are usually the most suitable, except where PMMA is necessary to provide a robust lens for handling. Myopia control is achieved with PMMA [1] and to a lesser extent with modern hard lenses [2], which are physiologically superior. Hard lenses may prove more acceptable after previous soft lens wear.

29.2.2 Hypermetropia

Strabismic children, especially those with accommodative esotropia, derive greatest benefit. Normal hypermetropes may find vision better with spectacles, but comments at school may initiate contact lens wear.

Soft lenses are the first choice for infants under 6 years and for most older children, depending on the degree of astigmatism, the acceptance of a hard lens, and sporting and other school activities.

29.2.3 Anisometropia

Unilateral myopes or hypermetropes, whether axial or refractive, may benefit from a combination of contact lens wear and part-time occlusion. Success is often greater than with spectacles, although in some cases they merely keep an amblyopic eye straight [3]. If extended wear is necessary with dense amblyopia, the risks outweigh the visual benefits and contact lenses are contraindicated.

29.3 Therapeutic applications

29.3.1 Aphakia

Early treatment and optical correction are essential for bilateral aphakic infants, so that contact lenses give significant long-term visual benefits [4]. Extended wear soft lenses may be used initially, but only as a prelude to daily wear because of the risk of infection. Hard lenses can be fitted with confidence for children over 5 years. Silicone can be used with success where soft lens loss is a major problem.

Typical specification

Baby (1–6 months) 75% water content   7.00/12.00 + 32.00 D
Infant (1–4 years)   60% water content   7.60/13.50 + 25.00 D
Child (5–10 years)   60% water content   7.80/14.00 + 15.00 D

Practical advice

- Over-correct babies for arm's length vision, which is the range of their visual world.
- Prescribe bifocal spectacles over the lenses for close work at school.

29.3.2 Albinism

Albinism is associated with nystagmus, ametropia (often with high astigmatism) and photophobia. A tinted hard lens is best, but often there is no visual improvement over spectacles. Tinted soft lenses are more comfortable and may well help infants.

Practical advice

- Carefully observe any nystagmus with hard lenses because it may increase with the stress of adaptation.

29.3.3 Aniridia and iris coloboma

These conditions require an opaque iris lens to occlude the light (*see* Section 24.2). Colour matching of the good eye is important at school, for psychological reasons.

29.3.4 Microphthalmos

Microphthalmic eyes are usually fitted for cosmetic rather than visual reasons. They tend to have steep corneal radii (e.g. 6.80 mm) with high hypermetropia (e.g. +10.00 D), so that aphakic design can be used with an arbitrary power of about

+10.00 D. Unilateral cases can be fitted with a tinted soft lens where the plus power makes the eye look larger. This is easier to fit and more comfortable than a scleral shell.

Practical advice

- A cosmetic lens for one disfigured eye is more often the parent's idea rather than the child's.
- Carefully consider the long-term effects, since a child often refuses to go out without the lens.

29.4 Non-therapeutic fitting

If a child is happy in spectacles, the parents are best dissuaded from the idea of contact lenses. However, they can sometimes be very successful as young as 7 years old, although 10–12 years is a more usual age to consider fitting. The following criteria apply:

- Visual correction is required all the time.
- The child wants lenses.
- The parents want the child to have lenses.
- The child is old enough to understand handling and maintenance.

Keratometry readings are in the same range as those for adults and the fitting technique is therefore the same. Aftercare is imperative because of the potential number of years lenses may be worn, and the material with the best physiological characteristics should be used.

The advantages and disadvantages of the various lens types are mainly as given in Section 3.3 but hard lenses are the probable first choice for myopes and high water content soft lenses for hypermetropes. Torics should initially be avoided because of the expense and risk of loss.

References

1. Stone, J. (1976) The possible influence of contact lenses on myopia. *British Journal of Physiological Optics*, **31**, 89–114
2. Perrigin, J., Perrigin, D., Quintero, S. and Grosvenor, T. (1990) Silicone-

acrylate contact lenses for myopia control: 3-year results. *Optometry and Vision Science*, **67**, 764–769
3. Morris, J. (1979) Contact lenses in infancy and childhood. *Contact Lens Journal*, **8**, 15–18
4. Taylor, D., Morris, J., Rogers, J.E. and Warland, J. (1979) Amblyopia in bilateral infantile and juvenile cataract. *Transactions of the Ophthalmological Society of the United Kingdom*, **99**, 170–176

Chapter 30

Therapeutic fitting with hard and soft lenses

Contact lenses are used for therapeutic reasons to:

- Correct vision in eyes with existing pathology.
- Correct irregular corneal astigmatism by providing a smooth optical surface.
- Promote healing by protecting denuded cornea and new epithelium from the lids.
- Prevent epithelial breakdown.
- Relieve pain or foreign body sensation.
- Protect the cornea and, when used in conjunction with lubricating solutions, provide a moist environment.

30.1 Aphakia

Unilateral aphakics derive considerable visual benefit from lenses because the reduced image size and lack of distortion allow some degree of both fusion and binocular vision to be established. The field of view is also considerably improved. Visual acuity, however, is often reduced by about one line because of the absence of spectacle magnification.

The key problems with aphakic contact lens wearers are:

- Different retinal image sizes.
- Handling difficulties.
- Centration problems.
- Pupil shape and flare.

30.1.1 Hard lenses

Hard and PMMA lenses give excellent visual results and are therefore the ideal optical correction for those able to handle lenses.

Corneal lens fitting

- The BOZR is often fitted between mean and steepest 'K' to help stability and centration and give the preferred fluorescein pattern of apical clearance.
- The BOZD is chosen between 7.00 mm and 8.50 mm, depending on pupil size and position.
- The TD is generally larger than with the equivalent low-powered lens to help centration; it varies between 8.80 mm and 10.50 mm.
- The peripheral curves are usually spherical. The axial edge lift is greater than normal, of the order of 0.15 mm.
- Lenses are lenticular in form to reduce weight and thickness. The FOZD is often 0.50 mm larger than the BOZD. 8.00 mm to 8.50 mm is fairly standard, depending on pupil shape and position and where the lens sits. The reduced optic varies inversely with power.
- The front peripheral curve is often in the form of a negative carrier, although parallel and even positive shapes are used.
- A typical centre thickness is 0.35–0.45 mm because of the high powers required.
- Peripheral fenestrations are often used with PMMA to help tears exchange. Central fenestrations can cause flare and visual disturbance.
- Edge thickness should be at least 0.16 mm to avoid a fragile 'knife edge' and make removal easier.

Practical advice

- Some high plus lenses always assume a decentred, superior temporal position because the corneal apex has been drawn in this direction during surgery. Choose the TD and BOZD to give sufficient pupil coverage for adequate vision.
- If lenses decentre down because of gravity and lens mass, fit larger ones.
- Use a negative carrier to give a 'hitch-up' lens.
- Avoid a back surface toric unless centration is a problem. Toric peripheries are sometimes necessary with high degrees of astigmatism.
- Tints reduce photophobia and assist handling; a different

density or colour between 'right' and 'left' helps identification.

● If exposed corneal sutures cause peripheral staining or are rubbed by the lens, they should be removed to enable comfortable wear. This may be necessary up to several months later.

Apex (corneoscleral) lens

The Apex is a very large, modified corneal lens with a scleral rim of about 2.00 mm and reduced optic to minimize mass [1,2]. It is a bicurve construction, with the peripheral curve at least 0.70 mm flatter than the BOZD. The lens is used where the corneal curvature is very flat in one meridian, grossly irregular or where an eccentric pupil requires a very large optic. The lenses give stable acuity because of their limited movement on the cornea and are especially useful for uniocular senile aphakics and also for grafted aphakic eyes. The wearing times can be reasonably long because of reduced corneal sensitivity.

● The BOZR is chosen approximately 0.50 mm flatter than 'K' to give apical touch.

● The BOZD varies from 8.00 mm to 9.50 mm to allow corneal alignment over a fairly large central area.

● The TD varies between 11.50 mm and 13.00 mm, depending on the corneal diameter. The large size assists handling.

● The lens periphery usually has up to six fenestrations.

Typical specification: 8.20:8.50/10.50:12.00 BVP +17.00 Tint 912

Practical advice

● Expect some degree of corneal staining because of the fitting technique.

● The wearing time may be limited, but even a few hours of good vision is appreciated if nothing else has worked.

It is important to ensure that the patient can handle the lens before ordering. Elderly aphakics often have loose lids, so removal is difficult. A suction holder is more useful if it incorporates a light source, but should only be used by patients who are aware of the lens position and can aim correctly. Bilateral aphakics can use a spectacle frame glazed on one side only. The help of a friend or relative is invaluable.

The success rate is greater with binocular cases, whereas young unilateral aphakics often find tolerance difficult with a hard lens. The cause is often traumatic and they find it difficult to appreciate the potential consequences of lost binocular vision, amblyopia and divergence. A comfortable hydrophilic lens often achieves greater success.

30.1.2 Soft lenses

Most major companies produce lenses in a range of water content in powers of +10.00 D to +20.00 D. Fitting criteria are mainly as given in Chapter 16.

Low water content lenses

Lenses may vary in size from 12.50 mm to 14.50 mm with BOZRs from 8.10 mm to 9.50 mm. The design is usually a bicurve construction, with FOZDs between 10.00 mm and 13.00 mm. A front surface aspheric (e.g. Allergan) minimizes centre thickness but makes handling more difficult.

The BOZR is chosen to be approximately 0.50 mm flatter than 'K' for corneal diameter lenses and from 0.70 mm to 1.30 mm flatter than 'K' for semi-scleral lenses.

Lens size must always be chosen to avoid the limbus and give good centration. Irregularities at the limbus such as sutures or drainage blebs influence the choice of diameter. Exposed sutures should be removed, while deformities at the limbus may need to be vaulted with a diameter as large as 16.00 mm.

Medium water content lenses

Lenses have TDs between 13.00 mm and 14.50 mm. BOZRs range from 7.80 mm to 9.30 mm and are chosen 0.50–1.00 mm flatter than 'K' for semi-scleral designs.

High water content lenses

Lenses are mainly semi-scleral bicurves, with BOZDs from 7.00 mm to 8.00 mm and TDs between 13.50 mm and 14.50 mm. 16.00 mm diameters are available from some small manufacturers. BOZRs range from 7.80 mm to 9.00 mm and are selected only about 0.3 mm flatter that 'K' for diameters up to 14.00 mm. The range is steeper than with lower water content lenses because the softer materials require fitting closer to 'K' to ensure stability.

Practical advice

● Try more than one lens design, because different makes can give very different acuities.

● Always over-refract with the type of lens to be used, since the BVP may vary by at least 1.00 D between different designs.

● Centration also varies with design and lenticulation.

Continuous wear (see also Chapter 20)

Elderly aphakics who are unable to handle lenses may leave them in continuously. Careful practitioner management and regular aftercare visits are extremely important, since most documented infections associated with extended wear have been with this type of patient [3].

Lens movement is especially important because of overnight dehydration and the need to ensure the removal of debris. A saline eyewash in the morning and evening can be recommended, ideally using minims. Deposits are a major problem and some patients need a new lens every 3–6 months.

30.2 Keratoconus

Keratoconus is the classic case in which a hard contact lens provides a new refracting surface for an irregular cornea and gives good acuity where spectacles are unable to manage adequate improvement. Corneal lenses are the preferred form of correction in the early stages of the condition.

The apex of the cone is usually displaced inferior and nasal relative to the pupil. The common problem in all keratoconus fitting is to make the BOZD of the lens, which tends to centre at the apex of the cone, sufficiently large to cover the pupil area without the formation of either dimples or a stagnant pool of tears.

Keratometry readings are typically steep, astigmatic and irregular, except in the early stages. As the cone advances, readings eventually fall outside the range of the instrument, although this can be extended with a supplementary plus lens (*see* Section 2.2.4).

The main problems with keratoconus fitting are:

- Decentration on the irregular cornea.
- Discomfort because of increased lid and corneal sensitivity.
- Photophobia (helped by a tint).
- Lens thickness because of the high negative power.
- Dimpling which may necessitate fenestrations or a change in peripheral design.
- Oedema, often due to lack of lens mobility and reduced tears exchange.

30.2.1 Hard lenses

Spherical lenses to give 'three-point touch'

- The BOZR is chosen on or near the flattest 'K'.
- The BOZD is between 5.00 mm and 7.00 mm.
- The TD ranges from 8.50 mm to 9.50 mm.
- The peripheral curves are designed to flatten off rapidly to follow the topography of the cornea.
- When the patient is using the cone area, the BVP is usually much higher minus than expected because of the steep BOZR. In advanced cases, the patient may use the periconal area and require less power.

The optimum 'three-point touch' fluorescein fit (Figure 30.1) gives the overall effect of a 'bulls-eye' pattern. There is touch on

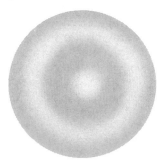

Figure 30.1 Typical 'bull's-eye' fluorescein pattern (dark shading represents the fluorescein)

the cone surrounded by a ring of fluorescein which is in turn surrounded by an annulus of mid-peripheral bearing with peripheral edge clearance. If the central touch is too heavy, it may allow rocking of the lens and cause corneal abrasion. This can be improved either by changing the BOZR or by altering the degree of peripheral bearing.

Typical trial lenses [4]:

5.50:5.60/6.50:7.60/8.50:8.60   −11.00
6.50:6.00/7.50:8.00/9.50:9.00   −5.50
7.00:6.00/8.00:8.20/10.00:9.20   −3.00

The rule that a radius change of 0.05 mm ≡ 0.25 D breaks down because of the very steep curves.

Rule of thumb

A change in radius of 0.05 mm ≡ 0.50 D with lenses steeper than 6.90 mm.

Rule of thumb

Select the initial BOZD to be approximately equal to the BOZR + 0.20 mm (e.g. 7.40 mm with 7.20 mm radius; 6.20 mm with 6.00 mm radius).

Spherical lenes to fit the corneal periphery

In fairly early keratoconus, especially with large corneas, lenses can be fitted on the basis of matching the relatively unchanged corneal periphery [5] but with the addition of a much steeper BOZR. The actual peripheral curves are very similar to those found in a lens designed for a normal cornea, but to allow for the steep centre a tricurve becomes a four- or possibly five-curve lens.

Examples
'K'   6.60 mm along 170° × 6.10 mm along 65°
   central fitting   peripheral fitting
   6.75:7.00/   7.80:7.70/8.60:8.50/10.50:9.50

'K' 6.60 mm along 50°   other meridian off the scale
central fitting   peripheral fitting
6.90:7.10/7.70:7.60/   8.50:8.20/9.30:9.00/10.50:10.00
'K' 6.25 mm along 65:   other meridian off the scale
central fitting   peripheral fitting
6.50:6.80/7.20:7.40/   8.20:8.20/9.00:9.00/10.50:9.60/12.25:10.00

Offset and aspheric lenses

These designs have the advantage that, if the conical zone of the cornea lies in front of the visual axis, a small diameter lens can be fitted.

- The BOZR is chosen on flattest 'K' to give an area of central touch.
- The BOZD varies from 2.00 mm for a true conoid to 7.70 mm for some offsets.
- The TD is typically 8.00 mm, but may be as small as 7.00 mm.
- Axial edge lift is the standard 0.10–0.15 mm and assessed by fluorescein.
- Fenestrations may be used to improve tears exchange and reduce frothing.

Typical offset trial lens [6]: 6.00:5.50/AEL (ff) 0.1 at 8.50.

Elliptical 'K' (Persecon E)

The design has a bi-elliptical back surface and works well for early keratoconus, especially where patients have large pupils [7].

- The BOZR is chosen on flattest 'K'.
- The optic zone is 8.00–8.50 mm, allowing an even pressure distribution over the lens centre.
- The TD is either 9.30 mm or 9.80 mm.
- The eccentricity of 0.39 is the same as that of the standard Persecon E (*see* Section 10.2).
- The peripheral zone flattening has an elliptical curve of the same eccentricity but flatter vertex radius [8].

The design is predetermined by the laboratory, so that if the fluorescein pattern is unsatisfactory another type of fitting should be used.

Practical advice

- Do not fit too steep as this may result in a large air bubble.
- The steeper the radius, the higher the minus power.
- Small changes in BOZR can give larger than expected changes in refraction.
- Modifying peripheral curves can affect the lens position and the required BVP.
- Even if the first trial lens is not ideal, over-refract to get an idea of the likely acuity. It is always better to assess the vision with at least two trial lenses.
- Lens design may depend on visual improvement.
- Expect to use at least two lenses per eye.
- The first lens can be made in PMMA and the final lens in a modern material.
- Sometimes a high *Dk* material is less comfortable than a low *Dk* material.
- Sometimes PMMA is the most comfortable of all.
- PMMA is more stable and can be made thinner.

30.2.2 Soft lenses

Soft lenses can sometimes be used for keratoconus, depending upon the degree of corneal distortion. Centre thickness is deliberately increased or a conical back surface used.

Spherical soft lenses

The minimum centre thickness should be 0.35 mm, but 0.60 mm is advisable. The edge is reduced to 0.18 mm by means of lenticulation. A relatively rigid +5.00 D HEMA lens masks a considerable degree of corneal distortion and reasonable acuity may be obtained with the additional use of spectacles.

Trapezoid lenses

The trapezoid lens is designed to vault the conical area of the cornea [9]. The back surface has a central portion between 11.00 mm and 15.00 mm in radius, with a steeper peripheral curve of 8.50 mm. The TD is 15.00 mm, and a third curve of radius 9.50 mm is introduced if the edge is too tight.

The lenses are made in HEMA for rigidity, with a centre thickness of 0.60 mm and low plus power. Some degree of corneal moulding occurs, but it is less than with a conventional lens. The fitting depends on the size and steepness of the cone and should be assessed with a trial lens.

Example:
HEMA trapezoid trial lens:
12.00:8.50/8.00:14.00/9.00:15.00   +5.00 D t_c 0.60 mm

Scleral soft lenses

A multicurve soft scleral lens with a diameter of 23.00 mm can be designed from a mould of the eye using a shadowgraph.

30.3 Corneal grafts (keratoplasty)

30.3.1 Hard lenses

The main considerations are:

● The size of the graft. It is better to keep the TD within the limits of the graft tissue.

● The tilt of the graft, which may cause a problem in position and stability. Lens decentration often occurs but is acceptable if the graft is not compromised.

● Stability. Sometimes a very large lens (>12.00 mm) is necessary even to stay on the cornea with blinking.

● Staining of the grafted tissue is less acceptable than with normal cornea and requires careful observation. Any coalescent areas are unacceptable.

Examples:
Offset 1   7.60:6.50/AEL (ff) 0.10 at 8.50
Apex   7.80:8.00/10.50:12.50

30.3.2 Soft lenses

A soft bandage lens can compress or mould a low rigidity graft or realign a partially everted graft and is often used as a protective membrane immediately the sutures have been inserted. Soft lenses are also used to treat graft rejection. The soft 'splint' is often kept in place for several weeks.

30.4 Corneal irregularity

30.4.1 Hard lenses

The initial lens is chosen on the basis of the best keratometry readings obtainable. The lens is fitted in the normal way, but the fluorescein pattern nearly always shows the irregularity of the corneal surface. The fitting is decided according to visual improvement. In some cases a small amount of apical clearance gives stability and good vision, whereas in others alignment or touch is necessary. The TD may need to be larger than normal for lens stability.

Bubbles over an irregular area can cause long-term corneal desiccation and may ultimately require a scleral lens.

30.4.2 Soft lenses

Soft lenses usually conform too closely to the cornea to give any great optical benefit. Some improvement is occasionally achieved with a thick lens or rigid material (e.g. CSI).

30.5 High myopia and hypermetropia

30.5.1 Hard lenses

The main problem with powers over $+10.00\,D$ is the lens mass. Stability and position may be improved by fitting:

- A TD about 0.50 mm larger than usual.
- On mean 'K' to show apical clearance with the fluorescein pattern.
- Lid attachment (hitch-up) lenses (*see* Section 6.5).
- A reduced optic and ordering the optimum design of carrier (e.g. parallel for a high minus with tight lids; negative for high plus).

30.5.2 Soft lenses

The main difficulty with myopes is the mass of material at the limbus. Even with a reduced optic, long-term problems such as oedema and vascularization can arise. The size of the optic is important: HO3 and HO4 lenses (Bausch and Lomb) have a large optic and greater average thickness, whereas CSI (Pilkington) have a small optic and more satisfactory thickness. The highest power normally available is −22.00 D which is equivalent to −35.00 D in spectacle form.

Hypermetropes, on the other hand, have all the lens mass centrally. This can cause central oedema even with high water content materials. A normal cornea is under greater stress than an aphakic eye because it has higher oxygen demands.

Radii are chosen in the normal way, but larger overall sizes are necessary to aid stability.

Practical advice

- Use a trial lens close to the anticipated power to give an accurate assessment of both BVP and fitting.
- Ensure that the back and front surface designs are consistent when replacing a lens to avoid visual and fitting difficulties.

30.6 Albinos

Hard lenses do not always give visual improvement despite frequently heavy and restrictive spectacles for bilateral hypermetropic astigmatism. Magnification is lost by fitting a contact lens and the cylinder gives unstable vision. The main benefit of contact lenses is to help photophobia by means of a tint and occasionally soft lenses may also be used (see Chapter 24). Adaptation is a stressful period and any nystagmus can increase initially, although it tends to stabilize once the lenses have settled down. Nystagmus sometimes reduces where vision is improved.

30.7 Radial keratotomy

Radial keratotomy is an invasive surgical technique to reduce myopia [10]. It changes the shape factor of the elliptical cornea from positive towards negative, so that it has a flat centre and steep periphery. Conventional trial lenses therefore show excessive edge clearance. Much tighter peripheral curves must be used or a laboratory design chosen with minimum edge clearance (e.g. Hanita Elliptical). The apical cap of the central cornea is also wider, so a large BOZD is needed for lens stability.

Example:

'K'   9.16 along 170°   8.71 along 80°

Redesigned tricurve lens [11]: 9.00:8.00/10.00:10.00/11.00:12.50

Hard lenses are more acceptable than soft because of the risks of vascularization and infection. PMMA should be avoided, as problems may arise with oedema and corneal warpage.

Visual and fitting complications occur as a result of the shape of the eye, diurnal variations in corneal shape and the patient's psychological state.

References

1. Fraser, J.P. and Gordon, S.P. (1967) The 'apex' lens for uniocular aphakia. *Ophthalmic Optician*, **7**, 1190–1253
2. Bagshaw, J., Gordon, S.A.P. and Stanworth, A. (1966) A modified corneal contact lens: binocular single vision in unilateral aphakia. *British Orthoptic Journal*, **23**, 19–30
3. Carpel, E. and Parker, P. (1985) Extended wear aphakic contact lens fitting in high risk patients. *Contact Lens Association of Ophthalmologists Journal*, **11**, 231–233
4. Woodward, E.G. (1989) Contact lenses in abnormal ocular conditions – keratoconus. In *Contact Lenses*, A.J. Phillips and J. Stone (eds), Butterworths, London, pp. 748–757
5. Shephard, A.W. (1989) Keratoconus contact lens fitting. *Journal of the British Contact Lens Association* (Scientific Meetings 1989) pp. 21–25
6. Ruben, M. (1975) *Contact Lens Practice*, Baillière-Tindall, London, pp. 283–284
7. Astin, C. (1987) Fitting of keratoconus patients with bi-elliptical contact lenses. *Journal of the British Contact Lens Association*, **10**, 24–28
8. Achatz, M., Eschmann, R., Rockert, H., Wilken, B. and Grant, R. (1985) Keratoconus – a new approach using bi-elliptical contact lenses. *Optometry Today*, **25**, 581–586
9. Ruben, M. (1978) *Soft Contact Lenses*, Baillière-Tindall, London, pp. 256–260
10. Fyodorov, S.N. and Durnev, V.V. (1979) Operation of dosaged dissection of corneal circular ligament in cases of myopia of mild degree. *Annals of Ophthalmology*, **11**, 1885
11. Astin, C. (1986) Contact lenses for patients after radial keratotomy. *Transactions of the Annual Clinical Conference of the British Contact Lens Association*, **3**, 2–7

Chapter 31

Other lenses for therapeutic fitting

31.1 Scleral lenses

Visual indications

- Ocular topography makes corneal lens fitting difficult.
- Eccentric pupils.
- Where a high powered corneal or soft lens fails to centre.

Protective indications

- Tears retention in some dry eye conditions (e.g. Stevens–Johnson syndrome, Sjögren's syndrome).
- Corneal exposure (e.g. inadequate lid closure, exophthalmic precorneal tear film failure).
- Fornix support (e.g. following reconstruction surgery, alkali burn).
- Entropion and trichiasis.
- Protection for anaesthetic cornea.
- Occlusion.
- Ptosis.

Fitting indications

- Poor centration with other designs.
- Poor stability with a corneal lens.

Impression fitting is the preferred method because it can deal with virtually any eye. Subsequent lens modifications are made according to the specific condition.

A ptosis prop is made by using a shelf-type support by cutting through the full thickness of a 2–3 mm thick shell [1].

In symblepharon, a hard scleral ring can be used. This is

usually 4 mm wide and is effectively the scleral portion without the optic.

31.2 Combination lenses

31.2.1 'Piggy-back' lenses

The combination of a hard lens on top of a soft lens is used with keratoconus and graft cases to achieve good vision with improved comfort where all else has failed [2].

The foundation soft lens has a large diameter for stability and a typical front surface radius of about 7.60 mm. This is achieved by altering the power of the best fitting, so that a minus lens is necessary for 'K' readings between 6.00 mm and 7.00 mm. A low plus lens is required if the cornea is flatter than 8.00 mm.

The hard lens has a TD of 9.50 mm or larger to give good centration. The BOZR is based on the front surface curvature of the soft lens, measured with the keratometer.

The problems with combination lenses are:

- An extensive trial set of large steep soft lenses is required to find a satisfactory fitting.
- Stabilizing the hard lens on the soft takes practice.
- Different solutions are needed for each part of the combination.
- Lenses are removed separately. In some cases, the soft part is used for extended wear with the hard lens put in place to help vision during the day.

The reverse combination of a corneal hard lens covered by a thin soft lens is used for sporting purposes.

31.2.2 Hard centre with soft periphery

This combination (e.g. Softperm) is designed to give the acuity of hard lenses with the comfort of soft.

The hard central portion has a diameter of 8.00 mm and is made from synergicon A material. The soft peripheral flange has a diameter of 14.30 mm. The basic fittings consist of radii from 7.10 mm to 8.10 mm in 0.1 mm steps and the first choice of lens is near to flattest 'K'. Fitting characteristics of movement and centration are based on soft lens criteria [3]. Large molecular weight fluorescein can be used.

Problems prior to Softperm were:

- The soft skirt detaching from the hard centre.
- Bubbles often forming at the hard soft transition not eliminated by a change in fitting.
- Lenses fitting tightly to the eye, making removal difficult.
- The solutions must be compatible with both hard and soft lenses. Peroxide is now recommended.
- The low Dk of current materials.

31.3 Silicone lenses

Silicone lenses (*see* Section 5.4) have the following therapeutic uses [4]:

- Aphakia.
- Dry eyes, especially following therapy.
- Exposure problems following lid reconstruction.
- Corneal perforations.
- Corneal ulceration.

Trial sets consist of radii from 7.40 mm to 8.40 mm, with diameters from 11.70 mm to 13.20 mm in 0.50 mm steps (Wöhlk) and 10.80 mm (Danker). A wide range of powers is available, including plano and aphakic.

ADVANTAGES

- Very high Dk permits continuous wear.
- Good vision.
- They do not dehydrate and are ideal for dry eyes or tear film problems.
- Low risk of loss or damage.
- Good for corneal reconstruction. The radius can be refitted as the cornea reforms under the lens.
- Resistance to bacterial colonization and therefore ideal for eyes open to infection.
- They do not absorb foreign substances, so medication can be used without fear of contamination.
- Fluorescein can be used to ensure the optimum fitting.

DISADVANTAGES

- Difficult to fit.

- Surfaces deposits. Six-monthly replacements are advisable.
- Lenses can be difficult to remove.
- Adhesion can occur with lenses fitted either too steep or too flat.
- Expensive.

31.4 Bandage lenses

Soft bandage lenses are used on an extended wear basis to relieve pain and allow denuded epithelium to regain its normal structure. They are available in high or low water contents and are usually of plano power, since they are not primarily intended for visual improvement. Lenses are not generally handled by the patient and may require replacing every 4–8 weeks because of deposits. They are ideally fitted from stock and are used in cases of:

- Chronic keratitis.
- Post-keratoplasty.
- Bullous keratopathy.
- Exposure keratitis.
- Recurrent erosions.

31.4.1 General considerations

- Low water content is better where there is a tear film problem because it dehydrates less (e.g. exposure keratitis).
- High water content is better where a painful eye needs several weeks of continuous wear (e.g. bullous keratopathy).
- 'K' readings are not usually possible. A good starting point with a high water content lens is 8.50:14.50.
- Radii range from 7.80–9.50 mm, the flatter lenses often being made in the higher water content materials.
- Diameters vary between 13.50 mm and 16.50 mm, the larger lenses being made in the higher water content materials.
- Centre thickness varies between 0.10 mm and 0.25 mm, the lower water content lenses being thinner.
- Some lenses such as the Plano T (Bausch and Lomb) are 'one-fit'.

31.5 Additional therapeutic uses

DRUG-RELEASE LENSES

Soft lenses or shields of a collagen material are used as a drug-release mechanism [5].

LOW VISION AID

A Galilean telescope can be of benefit to the low-vision patient, but its cosmetic appearance is improved by using a high minus contact lens as the eyepiece. The powers required to achieve a minimum ×1.5 magnification are at least −25.00 D for the contact lens and +20.00 D for the spectacle lens. The problems are that the field of view reduces as the powers increase, and movement of the contact lens causes apparent movement of the visual field. However, the technique has been used with occasional success [6,7].

References

1. Trodd, T.C. (1971) Ptosis props in ocular myopathy. *Contact Lens*, **5**, 3–5
2. Westerhout, D.I. (1973) The combination lens and therapeutic uses of soft lenses. *Contact Lens Journal*, **4**, 3–22
3. Astin, C. (1985) Saturn II lenses and penetrating keratoplasty. *Transactions of the British Contact Lens Association Annual Clinical Conference*, **2**, 2–5
4. Woodward, E.G. (1984) Therapeutic silicone rubber lenses. *Journal of the British Contact Lens Association*, **7**, 39–40
5. Weissman, B. and Lee, D. (1988) Oxygen transmissibility, thickness and water content of three types of collagen shields. *Archives of Ophthalmology*, **106**, 1706
6. Silver, J.H. and Woodward, E.G. (1978) Driving with a visual disability – case report. *Ophthalmic Optician*, **18**, 794–795
7. Speedwell, L. (1986) 'Yet it does move': a successful and inadvertent Galilean telescopic system. *Optometry Today*, **26**, 109

Appendix

Vertex conversion table

Spectacle lens power	Vertex distance (mm)							
	Plus lenses				Minus lenses			
	8	10	12	14	8	10	12	14
4.00	4.12	4.12	4.25	4.25	3.87	3.87	3.87	3.75
4.50	4.62	4.75	4.75	4.75	4.37	4.25	4.25	4.25
5.00	5.25	5.25	5.25	5.37	4.75	4.75	4.75	4.62
5.50	5.75	5.75	5.87	6.00	5.25	5.25	5.12	5.12
6.00	6.25	6.37	6.50	6.50	5.75	5.62	5.62	5.50
6.50	6.87	7.00	7.00	7.12	6.12	6.12	6.00	6.00
7.00	7.37	7.50	7.62	7.75	6.62	6.50	6.50	6.50
7.50	8.00	8.12	8.25	8.37	7.12	7.00	6.87	6.75
8.00	8.50	8.75	8.87	9.00	7.50	7.37	7.25	7.35
8.50	9.12	9.25	9.50	9.62	8.00	7.87	7.75	7.62
9.00	9.75	9.87	10.12	10.37	8.37	8.25	8.12	8.00
9.50	10.25	10.50	10.75	11.00	8.87	8.62	8.50	8.37
10.00	10.87	11.12	11.37	11.62	9.25	9.12	8.87	8.75
10.50	11.50	11.75	12.00	12.25	9.62	9.50	9.37	9.12
11.00	12.00	12.37	12.75	13.00	10.12	9.87	9.75	9.50
11.50	12.62	13.00	13.37	13.75	10.50	10.37	10.12	9.87
12.00	13.25	13.62	14.00	14.50	11.00	10.75	10.50	10.25
12.50	13.87	14.25	14.75	15.25	11.37	11.12	10.87	10.62
13.00	14.50	15.00	15.50	16.00	11.75	11.50	11.25	11.00
13.50	15.12	15.62	16.12	16.62	12.25	11.87	11.62	11.37
14.00	15.75	16.25	16.75	17.50	12.62	12.25	12.00	11.75
14.50	16.50	17.00	17.50	18.25	13.00	12.62	12.37	12.00
15.00	17.00	17.75	18.25	19.00	13.37	13.00	12.75	12.37
15.50	17.75	18.25	19.00	19.75	13.75	13.50	13.00	12.75
16.00	18.25	19.00	19.75	20.50	14.25	13.75	13.50	13.00
16.50	19.00	19.75	20.50	21.50	14.50	14.12	13.75	13.50
17.00	19.75	20.50	21.50	22.25	15.00	14.50	14.12	13.75
17.50	20.50	21.25	22.25	23.25	15.37	14.87	14.50	14.00
18.00	21.00	22.00	23.00	24.00	15.75	15.25	14.74	14.37
18.50	21.75	22.75	23.75	25.00	16.12	15.62	15.12	14.75
19.00	22.50	23.50	24.75	26.00	16.50	16.00	15.50	15.00

Dioptre to millimetre conversion table   n = 1.336

36.00–9.37	40.12–8.41	44.25–7.63	48.37–6.98	52.50–6.43
36.12–9.34	40.25–8.38	44.37–7.61	48.50–6.96	52.62–6.41
36.25–9.31	40.37–8.36	44.50–7.58	48.62–6.94	52.75–6.40
36.37–9.27	40.50–8.33	44.62–7.56	48.75–6.92	52.87–6.38
36.50–9.24	40.62–8.30	44.75–7.54	48.87–6.91	53.00–6.36
36.62–9.21	40.75–8.28	44.87–7.52	49.00–6.89	53.12–6.35
36.75–9.18	40.87–8.25	45.00–7.50	49.12–6.87	53.25–6.34
36.87–9.15	41.00–8.23	45.12–7.48	49.25–6.85	53.37–6.32
37.00–9.12	41.12–8.20	45.25–7.46	49.37–6.84	53.50–6.31
37.12–9.09	41.25–8.18	45.37–7.44	49.50–6.82	53.62–6.29
37.25–9.06	41.37–8.16	45.50–7.42	49.62–6.80	53.75–6.28
37.37–9.03	41.50–8.13	45.62–7.40	49.75–6.78	53.87–6.26
37.50–9.00	41.62–8.10	45.75–7.38	49.87–6.77	54.00–6.25
37.62–8.97	41.75–8.08	45.87–7.36	50.00–6.75	54.12–6.23
37.75–8.94	41.87–8.06	46.00–7.34	50.12–6.73	54.25–6.22
37.87–8.91	42.00–8.03	46.12–7.32	50.25–6.72	54.37–6.21
38.00–8.88	42.12–8.01	46.25–7.30	50.37–6.70	54.50–6.19
38.12–8.85	42.25–7.99	46.37–7.28	50.50–6.68	54.62–6.18
38.25–8.82	42.37–7.96	46.50–7.26	50.62–6.67	54.75–6.16
38.37–8.79	42.50–7.94	46.62–7.24	50.75–6.65	54.87–6.15
38.50–8.76	42.62–7.92	46.75–7.22	50.87–6.63	55.00–6.13
38.62–8.73	42.75–7.89	46.87–7.20	51.00–6.62	55.12–6.12
38.75–8.70	42.87–7.87	47.00–7.18	51.12–6.60	55.25–6.10
38.87–8.68	43.00–7.85	47.12–7.16	51.25–6.58	55.37–6.09
39.00–8.65	43.12–7.82	47.25–7.14	51.37–6.57	55.50–6.08
39.12–8.62	43.25–7.80	47.37–7.12	51.50–6.55	55.62–6.07
39.25–8.59	43.37–7.78	47.50–7.10	51.62–6.54	55.75–6.05
39.37–8.57	43.50–7.76	47.62–7.08	51.75–6.52	55.87–6.04
39.50–8.54	43.62–7.74	47.75–7.06	51.87–6.50	56.00–6.03
39.62–8.51	43.75–7.71	47.87–7.05	52.00–6.49	
39.75–8.49	43.87–7.69	48.00–7.03	52.12–6.47	
39.87–8.46	44.00–7.67	48.12–7.01	52.25–6.46	
40.00–8.43	44.12–7.65	48.25–6.99	52.37–6.44	

Index

313

318   Index